APPRECIATING MOM through THE LENS OF ALZHEIMER'S

A Care Giver's Story
— by Don Mesibov

Copyright © 2014 Don Mesibov
All rights reserved.
ISBN: 1495279227
ISBN 13: 9781495279225
Library of Congress Control Number: 2014901307
CreateSpace Independent Publishing Platform
North Charleston, South Carolina

Dedicated to the Ones I Love

To Susan and her mother, Ruth, whose strong love of family made these last nine months with Mom possible.

To Mom's grandchildren—Brian, Darren, Todd, Marli, and Raina—who gave to Mom in return for all she gave to us.

To my brother Gary, my cousin Gail, and to my late cousin Fred; the special bond of love and respect we share continues to support me and always will.

To Laurie Mesibov, Carole Homer, Diane and Lee Alexander, Leilani Fitzgerald, and the relatives and close friends who kept in touch and reminded us that we were not alone in what we saw and revered in Mom.

To Molly Mesibov, an editor of this manuscript, mother of our grandchildren, and daughter-in-law extraordinaire.

To Avery Rose Mesibov and Emelia Kathryn Mesibov, twins who will know their great-grandmother through what we can pass along and from what they can read about her in this book, as well as Mom's other great-grandchildren: Anna, Claire, Milo, Nell, and one as yet not named to be born to Molly and Darren in summer 2014.

SIX GREAT-GRANDCHILDREN

Mom passed away more than thirteen years ago; her first great-grandchild, Anna, was born eight months before her death, although Mom did not get to see her. Since then five more great-grandchildren have been born, with another due July 2014. Mom's legacy will be reflected in the people they become.

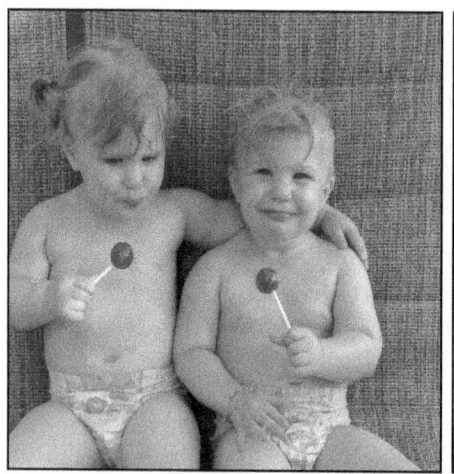

Avery Rose (left) and Emelia Kathryn, two years of age.

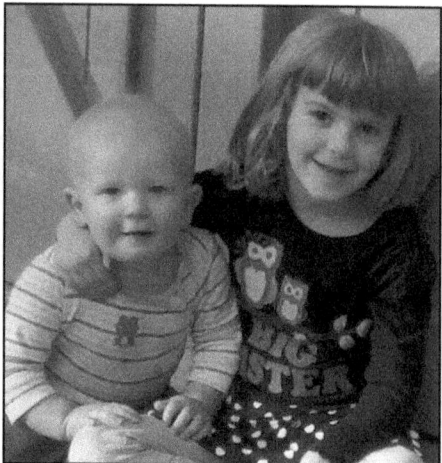

Milo (left) and Nel, early 2014

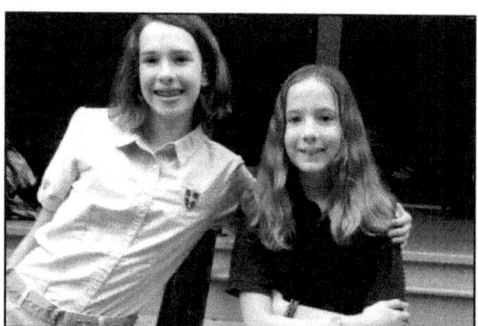

Anna (left) and Claire, January 2013.

Acknowledgments

A special acknowledgement to my wife, and the love of my life for thirty years, Susan Mesibov who has endured much ribbing (good natured, we think) for cajoling friends and relatives into poses and smiles as she has accumulated the thousands of pictures, since 1983, from which the majority of photos in this book have been selected. Susan has also been the primary editor and partner in the writing of this book. She read and reread drafts of the manuscript and continually located grammatical and spelling errors and highlighted passages that needed to be shortened, deleted or expanded upon.

While I am not proud of my technological shortcomings I am aware of them and this book would have been delayed a long time if not for Susan's technological assistance.

To those who labored through some of my earlier drafts and offered the suggestions and encouragement that allowed me to improve the manuscript from being a potential source of embarrassment to the point where I am no longer afraid to release it to the public: Carol Amberg, Chapin Dwyer, Alice Edelstein, Pat Flynn, Donna Halper, Adrienne Hartman, Barbara Kearns, Carole and Greg Littell, Fran Mesibov, and Jim Waterson.

In addition, an acknowledgement, with love, goes to two of the three people I have been closest to since our earliest childhood days. My brother Gary and my cousin Gail have been in constant communication with me supplying anecdotes, photos, and memories to supplement my own as well as reviewing and commenting on drafts of this manuscript. Writing this book brought back recollections of wonderful experiences we shared with each other and with Gail's brother, Fred, whom we lost in 2006.

About the Author

Don Mesibov is an author, journalist and professional educator whose portfolio showcases a wide variety of writing. He is co-author of three nonfiction books, including *Captivating Classes with Constructivism*, published by Rainmaker Education in 2013. He also co-authored two other titles on education published by Eye on Education in 2004.

Mesibov previously worked as a weekly newspaper reporter, editor, and middle school English teacher. Since 1998 he has been writing a weekly on-line column on issues in education that reaches approximately three thousand professional educators, parents and others interested in the field of education. He is also an adjunct professor in the education department of St. Lawrence University in Canton, New York, and is founder and director of the Institute for Learning Centered Education which has sponsored a week-long conference each summer since 1995 that models teaching strategies for actively engaging students in the learning process.

Currently, Mesibov continues to work as an educational consultant conducting workshops for teachers, administrators, parents and students that focus on how to make learning fun, challenging, and meaningful.

Contents

Chapter 1: The Move to a Retirement Home 1
Chapter 2: Ed Finally Admits It: "Mom Has Alzheimer's"............ 7
Chapter 3: Who Was Mom before Alzheimer's? 14
Chapter 4: A Father-and-Son Relationship................................. 25
Chapter 5: Mom Moves to Potsdam... 31
Chapter 6: Laughter and Pathos... 36
Chapter 7: Mom as Elwood P. Dowd... 55
Chapter 8: The Family Tree Sparks Memories........................... 65
Chapter 9: Rapid Deterioration: "I Wish I Could Die"................ 76
Chapter 10: Ten for Dinner... 98
Chapter 11: Mom Falls Four Times 109
Chapter 12: Mom's Life Gives the Universe Meaning 147
Chapter 13: A New Diagnosis: Four Weeks to Live 154
Chapter 14: The Patient Continues to Hold Her Own 176
Chapter 15: Simone, the Incompetent Caregiver....................... 190
Chapter 16: A Thief in Our Midst... 212
Chapter 17: Grandma, These Flowers Are for You 237

MOM ENJOYS HER GRANDCHILDREN

Mom had a smile for everyone, but for her grandchildren, it was always a bit brighter.

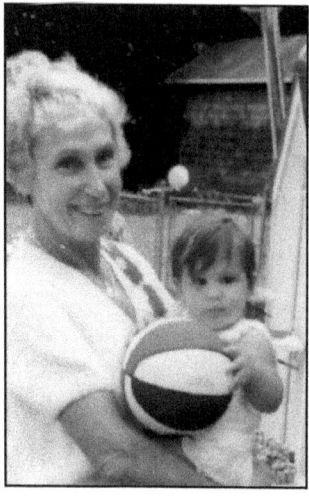

Mom holding Marli in 1987, when Marli was two years old.

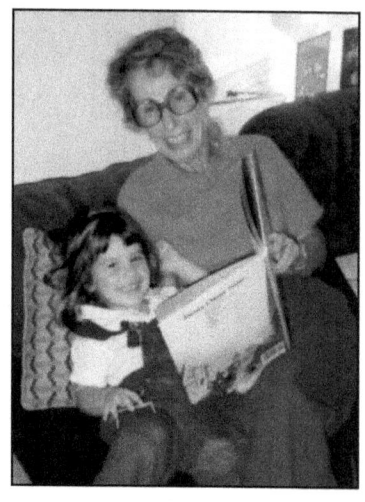

Reading to granddaughter Marli.

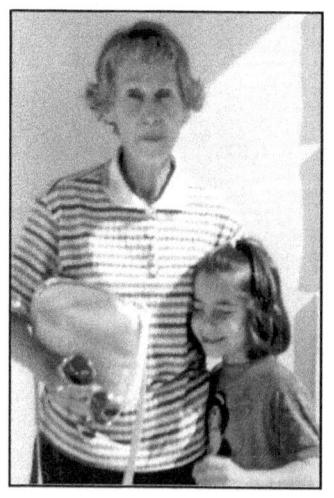

With granddaughter Raina, 1993, when Raina was three.

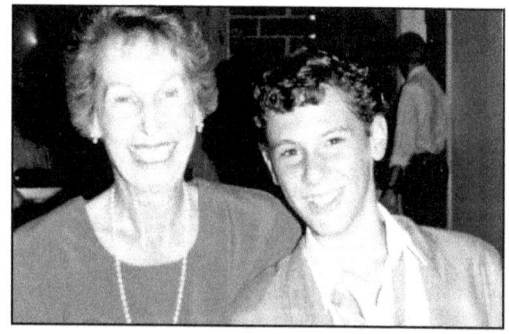

With grandson Darren, 1988, when he had just turned thirteen.

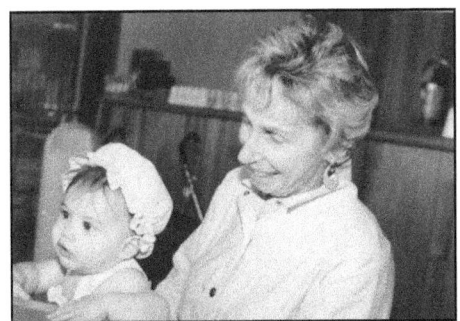

With Marli, as a baby, December, 1986.

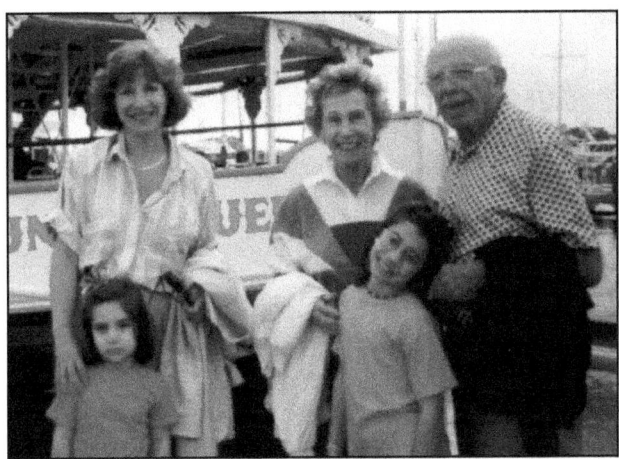

Mom and Ed take Raina, Marli, daughter-in-law Susan, and son Don on a dinner cruise during their visit to Florida, 1994.

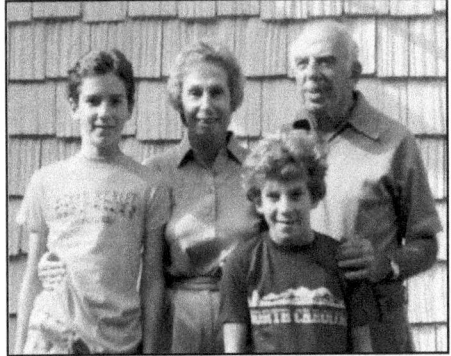

Mom and Ed pose with grandchildren Brian (left) and Todd, whose parents are Mom's younger son Gary and Laurie.

Chapter 1

The Move to a Retirement Home

We were fortunate. Even though Alzheimer's had steadily eroded Mom's recognition of us, her personality and ever-present smile were with her to the end. Her warmth and inquisitiveness remained her calling cards. I had heard that some Alzheimer's victims experience a dramatic change in personality—but not Mom. Growing up, the compliment I recall receiving from her most frequently was, "Donnie, you have a wonderful smile; always use it." And she modeled what she recommended to me.

The physical proximity to Mom that circumstances gave us near the end was wonderful for me and was one of the most meaningful experiences for our children and my wife, Susan. Mom contributed greatly to our personal growth at a time when she could not always recognize us and when she could not participate in a coherent conversation. She contributed by being Mom, maintaining so much of the personality of the person she'd previously been. While she had always been a caring, loving mother and doting grandmother, it was the last nine months of her life that had the greatest impact on me and on the memories I continue to cherish.

Susan and I had suspected that Mom might have Alzheimer's for at least two years prior to our August 2000 visit, which was when unforeseen circumstances enabled us to confirm our worst fears. Mom's repetition of questions that had been asked and answered earlier in the same telephone conversation had become increasingly difficult to ignore:

"Do you know when you and Susan will be down to visit? Larry (her husband, Ed's, son in Iowa) has asked about coming down at Christmastime with Dee and the children; is there any chance you would be coming then too?"

"No, Mom, we'll be down with Marli and Raina in February. It works better for us then, and this way you won't have to put up anyone in a motel. Also, Darren may be able to join us if we come in February. We've offered to fly him in from Flagstaff."

Five minutes later in the same conversation: "Donnie, will you and Susan be coming down around Christmastime this year?"

"No, Mom, we'll—"

But even years earlier, the clues were there for us to see—if there had been reason for us to look for them. Starting sometime in the early 1990s, Mom would occasionally go two weeks between routine phone calls to us. This might not be cause for taking notice in some families; however, since 1959 when I had left home for college, Mom's two o'clock Sunday phone calls had been a staple. The calls had continued through my 1983 marriage to Susan and had became much longer in duration when Susan was home to receive them since Susan usually gave Mom much more information about our lives than I offered. She also learned much more about Mom's and Ed's lives. On the rare occasion when Mom might be at a show or otherwise occupied at two o'clock on a Sunday, she would invariably call that night or, at latest, the next day. When she started to occasionally allow two weeks to go by between calls, this should have been a tip-off.

Another tip-off should have been in 1993 when Mom forgot to pass along to us a last-minute verbal invitation to a wedding and then didn't attend herself, even though it was a grandchild whom she adored. Ironically, we were actually visiting with Mom and Ed at their Florida home the day of the wedding, and we all could have easily attended if Mom had remembered to tell us about it. She subsequently explained that she had no recollection of being told of the invitation, and we chalked it up to miscommunication.

There were two other telltale signs that were so subtle I could only attribute them to her Alzheimer's long after she had passed. In the sixties and seventies, whenever friends would stop by to visit my first wife, Fran, and me, Mom would welcome an invitation to join us in the living room for coffee and talk. We would sometimes play a game, and at times she would come out to dinner with us. Her thorough enjoyment of these opportunities continued when Susan and I met and were then wed. Mom was so genuine in her conversations with our friends, so focused on learning about whomever she was with, and so obviously interested in what people were saying that she ingratiated herself with anyone she met.

I didn't think about it until a few years after her death, but in the late 1980s and thereafter, she would more often than not excuse herself if we had company when she was visiting. This was such a subtle change because with anyone else you might think that he or she was just being polite by leaving you to entertain your guests. However, this was unusual for Mom. She had always enjoyed meeting our friends and being in the company of people she didn't know very well. I guess I didn't give it much thought because I must have assumed that it was advancing age or being tired. However, as I've continued to read about people with Alzheimer's, I have become aware of their hesitancy to be in situations with anyone or anything that is not completely familiar. Perhaps Mom's withdrawal from the social situations she once relished was an indication of the onset of Alzheimer's years before her repetitious questions during phone calls made it obvious.

What could have been another equally subtle clue came in the late 1980s or early '90s, years before we had any reason to question whether anything was wrong with Mom. When I asked her "Do you ever bake apple pies anymore?" she told me that she didn't remember having baked apple pies, even after I said that they had been my favorite homemade treat and recalled having pleaded with her, as a child, to "please make another apple pie."

One reason it may have taken us so long to recognize the severity of Mom's dementia was the reaction of her husband of twenty-nine years when I had asked him a year earlier if there was any chance that Mom had Alzheimer's. Ed had been a general practitioner, and when I had asked whether she had the disease, he had told me unequivocally, "She does not have Alzheimer's—just a normal amount of memory loss that comes with aging."

May 2000

It was a three-year effort of ours—along with my brother Gary and sister-in-law Laurie—to convince Mom and Ed to sell their two-bedroom home in Royal Palm Beach, Florida. We wanted them to move the few miles to The Classic, a retirement home within a larger complex that included an assisted living section that they could ease into if it became necessary. We would have preferred that they move closer to either of our families. Gary had investigated locations in the Chapel Hill area, where he and Laurie lived; Susan had proposed building an addition onto our home. We all finally accepted the reality that it was difficult enough for them to consider a move from the home they had designed and had built in 1973. There was no way they would also be amenable to leaving the immediate area where they socialized with their remaining friends and held many memories.

For a long time, Mom and Ed resisted the thought of moving at all. They experienced the same trepidations that confront many retirees at a certain age. Most of their neighborhood friends had passed away or moved to live with or near their children. The maintenance of their house was more than they could handle. I would wince every time I saw Ed reach for a box from a high shelf in his garage—often standing on a ladder—knowing that one slip at his age could be fatal. Yet to my folks, this was still a place where my family and Gary's could visit, as would Ed's two children and his grandchildren. Who knew what else moving out of their home of nearly thirty years represented to them?

Finally, the decision was made; they signed a two-year contract with The Classic, and their home was put up for sale. Susan and I visited for a weekend to help them organize their possessions for the move to The Classic. Susan suggested an organizational strategy of going through the closets, cupboards, and shelves, placing all items in one of three piles in the main hallway:

- Definitely getting rid of,
- Giving to one of the children or grandchildren, and
- Definitely taking to the retirement home.

Initially the strategy appeared to be working. The four of us reviewed each item, and Mom and Ed agreed on the appropriate pile. The largest pile was the "definitely getting rid of" pile, and the smallest pile was for "definitely taking to the retirement home." But as Susan and I continued walking past the piles of items and rotating from room to room and back, we noticed that what started as the largest pile gradually began to shrink in size, while the pile of things they were definitely taking with them was increasing to the point of being impractically large. Each time Mom or Ed passed the "definitely getting rid of" pile, they had second thoughts and shifted an item or two out of that pile. After much piling and reorganizing, they moved at the end of June. We made plans for our next visit, with two of our three children, at the end of August.

Marli, now 28, reminisces about who Grandma was before Alzheimer's:
The one time I remember most being with Grandma was in Florida, "teaching" her to make lemonade. She had never made lemonade before, and she let me take control. I made her kitchen a mess, and the lemonade was absolutely undrinkable, but she gamely tasted each new batch and gave me her opinion on whether it needed still more sugar. I always looked forward to being with Grandma because she let me feel like I was teaching her. Most adults are constantly reminding children that the adults are in control. But Grandma asked my opinion on whether to wear sunscreen outside or how to make lemonade.

Laurie reminisces about her mother-in-law:
I recall the first time we visited her and Ed in Royal Palm Beach. This was just one of the many times when she seemed especially happy.

Appreciating Mom Through the Lens of Alzheimer's

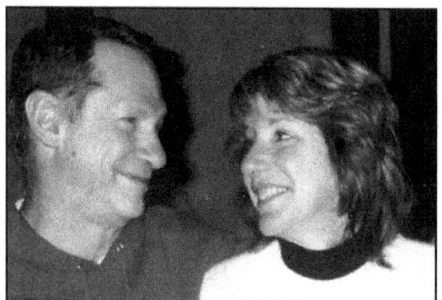 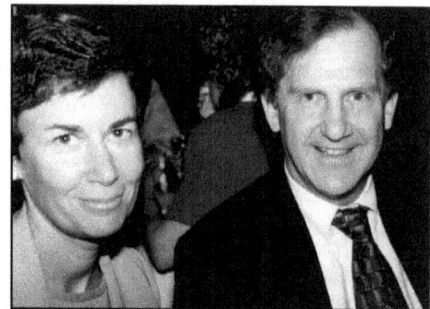

Mom's boys: Don next to his wife, Susan, and Gary alongside his wife, Laurie.

Chapter 2

Ed Finally Admits It: "Mom Has Alzheimer's"

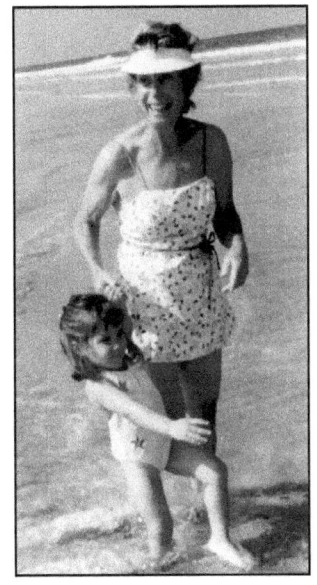

Mom at the beach with Marli (age two), near her home in Royal Palm Beach, Florida.

On Saturday, August 26, 2000, our daughters Marli, fifteen, and Raina, nine (almost ten), accompanied Sue and me for what we thought to be just another of our periodic visits to see Grandma and Grandpa. Our early morning flight from Syracuse, New York, to the West Palm Beach, Florida, airport was scheduled to take six hours, including a one-hour layover in Atlanta. We landed in Atlanta and found our way to the gate for our connecting flight, and I called home for messages. There was one on our answering machine from someone at The Classic, with a number for us to call upon arrival. Sue called immediately. A lady answered the phone and said that Ed had slipped in the shower last night, bruised some ribs, and was at the hospital. She said Mom was being taken care of, and that when we arrived we should go directly from the airport to the hospital, where we could meet Mom and see Ed.

In less than ten months, Mom and Ed would both be gone. But these months would be the most memorable and among the most wonderful of my life. It became an opportunity for us to experience who Mom was in a way that never would have happened if we had all, including Mom, continued to live our busy lives without the intimacy that was brought about by her Alzheimer's.

In our rental car, we went straight from the West Palm Beach Airport to the hospital, and Mom greeted us with her usual vibrant smile and warm hugs. "I'm so glad to see you and so worried about Ed," she said in the hospital waiting room. "How was your flight? Girls, you look great," she said to Marli and Raina. "How are you both doing?"

Ed, lying in the hospital bed, seemed his usual self. He asked us a few questions, greeted the grandchildren warmly, and alternately listened and dozed as the five of us gossiped and exchanged questions and stories—often with two or three of us disappearing into the lounge or to the cafeteria while the others stayed to keep Ed company. Ed's fall in the shower the night before resulted in internal bleeding. Prior to this event, he had been on doctor-prescribed Coumadin, which is defined on a website by the Cleveland Clinic, as "an anticoagulant (that) helps your body control how fast your blood clots; therefore, it prevents clots from forming inside your arteries, veins, or heart during certain medical conditions." This type of drug is often given to patients like Ed, who are at high risk for clotting in the arteries that supply blood to the brain. If a clot obstructs these arteries, it can cause a debilitating—if not fatal—stroke.

On the other hand, Ed's internal bleeding was exacerbated by the Coumadin and represented a serious threat to his life since clotting was needed to repair the internal damage and stop the bleed. This situation confronted his doctors with a dilemma that ultimately had no satisfactory resolution. Should the doctors take him off the Coumadin and risk a fatal blood clot, which would be much more likely given his condition, or should they continue him on the Coumadin and risk a fatal response due to an inability to stop the internal bleeding? It was a no-win choice. Ultimately they took him off the Coumadin, and it wasn't long after that he suffered a stroke. They then put him back on the blood thinner, and the internal bleeding resumed.

After spending less than twenty-four hours with Mom, we were certain of our amateur diagnosis of Alzheimer's, which was reinforced by Ed's own acknowledgement. Here—more than a year after his emphatic refusal to even consider that Mom might have Alzheimer's—lying in a hospital bed, he spoke of her condition as if that had always been his diagnosis. And maybe it had; perhaps he just hadn't wanted to acknowledge it to himself. But even then we didn't realize how far along it was until we started chauffeuring her to and from the hospital to visit Ed and sharing meals with her, usually at a restaurant near the hospital or in the hospital cafeteria.

Over the course of the next five days, before we returned to Potsdam to prepare the girls for the start of school, the degree of Mom's dementia manifested itself. Susan and I went shopping and left Marli and Raina with Grandma at her apartment at The Classic for a couple of hours. We returned to find Marli quite shaken. She told us that as Grandma walked them to the dining room in her retirement home someone approached and asked, "Are these your grandchildren?" Grandma responded, "No, I don't know who they are." "Grandma," Marli said, "we *are* your grandchildren." "Oh, of course you are!" Grandma responded.

It's hard to tell whether Ed knew that he would not leave the hospital alive or whether it was his usual pessimism coming to the fore (a nice complement to my mother's sometimes overdone optimism) when he called me to his side and said, "I'm worried about your mother. Please see that she's taken care of."

At another time, when he obviously thought he may be recovering, he pleaded that he didn't know how he could continue to take care of Mom. "Donnie, I can't take care of her anymore. It's become too much for me." Ed's physical condition eventually caused his death, but his mental acuity was as sharp at ninety-four as when I first met him when he was almost sixty-five, Mom was fifty-four, and I was thirty. As he lay in his hospital bed, he told us about the routines Mom would repeat many times each night before going to bed and the number of times she would wake him just to ask a nonsensical question or to repeat a question that she had asked and he had answered several times earlier in the day. He shared with us that during the last year they lived in their home, she had not cooked a meal because of the dangers due to her forgetfulness. We learned that they ate alone in The Classic dining room every night because even friends who used to join them for dinner couldn't handle Mom's inability to communicate and her circular conversations.

Susan was the first to explain to me why Mom had been able to hide from us the many symptoms that were so apparent now that we had spent such intimate time with her. "Ed covered for her a lot, and we didn't realize it," she said. "When she drives, Ed is always in the passenger seat next to her, telling her when to change lanes, when to turn, and where to brake. Think back to when we would go out to eat in recent years," Susan continued. "Mom would always wait for Ed to suggest what to order and then agree."

In past years they had frequently ordered two meals to share—a dining strategy they began when they were newlyweds in 1971—so none of us picked up on the fact that in the last few years it had always been Ed who had taken the lead in suggesting what to order. Ed would say, "Rhoda, why don't you order the chicken, I will get the salmon, and we'll share?"

After we had been out to eat with Mom several nights, Susan also noticed that Mom was always the last to order. "She doesn't have Ed to order for her, so she waits for us to order and then orders what you or I have ordered. That's why she ordered something spicy the other night even though we tried to remind her it was something she never ate because it would give her stomach problems. But it was what the previous person ordered, and she had developed the habit of ordering the last thing she heard."

Mom's inability to stay focused on the real world became apparent to me even more as we drove between The Classic and the hospital or the hospital and a restaurant as we waited out the times between visiting hours. Mom's speech was unaffected, and she could carry on a conversation for a while, but then she might say, "We'd better get home. Ed's probably there by now." I would respond, "Mom, Ed's still in the hospital; we have to get back there after lunch."

"Oh, okay," Mom would say. But then a minute later, "We'd better get home because Ed must be there by now." One time while we are riding in the car, she turned toward me and said, "Dad will be glad to see me. He's been gone all day." I thought she was referring to my first father, whom she always referred to as Dad when talking with me. I said, "Mom, Dad passed away many years ago. You're married to Ed now."

"I know who my husband is," she replied matter-of-factly, "but Dad always gets off the train around now and walks straight home." I realized that she was speaking of *her* father and situations that had occurred more than seventy years earlier. It occurred to me that Mom's inability to remain in the present might have a positive effect in the sense that she might not be able to feel the pain of Ed's illness and probable passing the way it would affect her if she were not suffering from this disease.

As it became apparent to us that Mom could not be left alone and that it was only Ed's constant presence that enabled her to give the appearance of independence, we spoke with the manager of The Classic. She recommended Alice, a lady who lived less than an hour away in Fort Lauderdale, as someone we could hire to be a live-in caregiver. Alice became invaluable to Mom throughout the month of September as someone who learned her routines, medications, and other needs.

When we left Royal Palm Beach after a five-day stay, Ed's son Larry and his wife, Dee, came down. We worked out a rotational shift through the end of September that assured us that either they, Gary, or our oldest child, Darren, who was twenty-five, would be with Mom and could transport her to the hospital every day. Over the years Gary's visits to Florida had been more frequent than ours, and he had been able to act as point person in our efforts to convince our folks to relocate to a home and find them a suitable place. The knowledge that he could quickly get from Chapel Hill to Royal Palm Beach in an emergency was reassuring to Susan and me because of the complexity of making connections from Northern New York, where the nearest major airport is almost a two-hour drive across the border in Canada. Gary offered to make regular visits over the next month if Ed's hospital stay extended into October. I indicated that either Susan or I would get down when possible, and we agreed to coordinate with Larry, Dee, and Darren so that we could each take on what we felt we could juggle along with our other family and work obligations. We compared schedules through November and were able to assure coverage for Mom for whatever length of time Ed was hospitalized—or hopefully, was back home but might still need outside assistance.

Brian reminisces about his grandmother:
I recall eating breakfast on her back porch, with fresh-squeezed orange juice. Enjoying being with her is what I remember most.

Raina reminisces about her grandmother:
If I were to sum up who Grandma was in one word, it would be "happy."

Ed Finally Admits It: "Mom Has Alzheimer's"

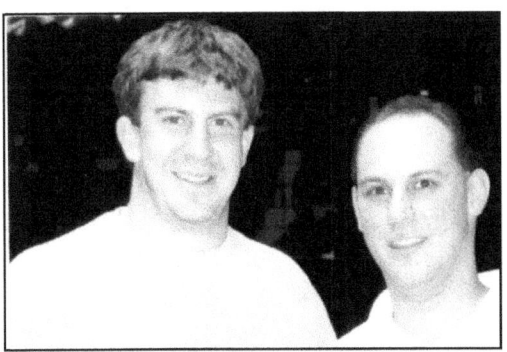

Grandchildren Todd (left) and Darren, born a month apart in 1975.

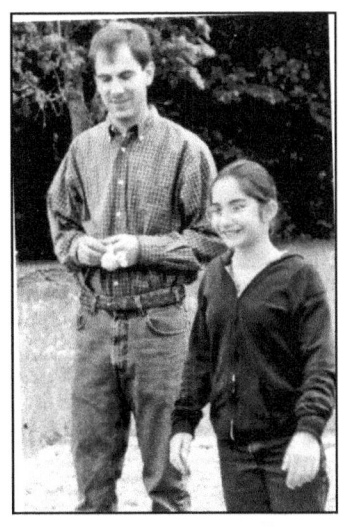

Grandchildren Brian and Raina in the late 1990s.

Chapter 3

Who Was Mom before Alzheimer's?

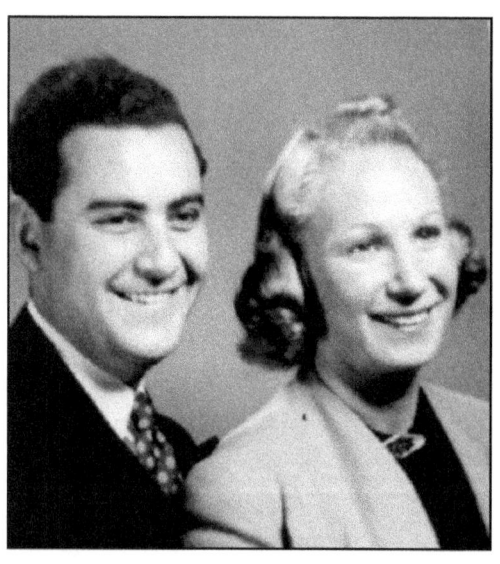

Mom with her first husband, Harold Mesibov, to whom she was married from September 3, 1938 until his death July 30, 1966. This picture was taken early in their marriage.

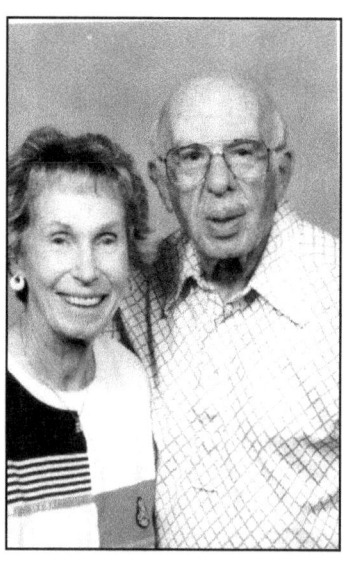

Mom with her second husband, Ed Meister, to whom she was married from May 15, 1971 until his passing, September 28, 2000.

Mom was fortunate to have had two wonderful marriages of twenty-eight and twenty-nine years, respectively. My natural father, Harold Mesibov, passed away July 30, 1966. He was fifty-two years old, the victim of a heart attack on a Maryland golf course only a few miles from their home. He was standing near the thirteenth green, waiting for his turn to putt.

I doubt that Mom and Ed would have been right for each other when they were younger. While Ed and his wife, from whom he had been widowed, raised wonderful children, Ed seemed more aloof than my dad. I don't think he and Mom would have clicked as a child-rearing couple. Gary sums it up best with a quote from Margaret Mead: "Every woman should have three husbands: one in their 20s to be madly in love with and have wild sex with; one in their 30s and 40s to be the father of their children and help to raise them; and one after 50 for companionship."

Mom and Dad were truly in love, having met while in their teens. Dad was the ideal partner for the child-rearing part, and Ed gave Mom companionship. In turn, Mom probably gave Ed an extra twenty years or more on his life. At her urging Ed took up golf, just to have a way of exercising together. They rarely kept score. If Mom hit a bad shot, rather than get frustrated, she was apt to pick up the ball and move it closer to the hole or even on to the next tee. As we got to know Ed, we grew to love him and to appreciate how perfect he was for Mom at this stage of her life.

They walked together every morning, played bridge with friends regularly, and had subscriptions to local theater offerings. They enjoyed dinners out with family and friends from up north (who were frequent visitors) as well as early bird specials with local friends.

Gary recollects the kind of person Mom was with the example that if she went into the ladies' room at a restaurant, she would emerge knowing about the lives and personalities of anyone who happened to be there. She was curious about people and preferred to ask questions even more than responding to them.

Similarly, my former wife, Fran, recalls a train ride to New York City: "You and I were seated next to each other, and your mother was sitting next to a stranger. She kept peppering this newfound friend with questions, as she did almost anyone she was with—particularly if it was the first time they had met. What was unique about Rhoda was that she was really interested in the responses she'd get to her questions. The evidence of her interest was that each time this stranger answered one of her questions, your mother's follow-up question would directly relate to what she had just heard.

"Your mother often asked me one question after another, and by the end of a conversation, I would realize that I had done most of the talking. I always came away from speaking with your mother feeling like, 'That was fun!' She was outgoing in such a one-on-one style—not outgoing in the sense of someone who can walk into a crowded room and capture the attention of everyone. I adopted your mother as a role model. What was special about her was that she cared about whoever she was with, and she sought out situations where she could learn as much as possible about someone. That never came easily to me, so I wanted to copy her approach. In a large group, she might rarely say a word, but she would seek out people she could talk with individually."

Physically, Mom was attractive but not an imposing figure. I read in an Associated Press article that "belly fat increases the risk of dementia." The article began, "Having a big belly in your 40s can boost your risk of getting Alzheimer's disease or other dementia decades later, a new study suggests." If the study is accurate, then Mom was an exception. Except for her two pregnancies, her five-foot figure barely carried more than a hundred pounds at its heaviest. But studies predict probability, and maybe this study was accurate for many people—but not all.

Mom played basketball at Lynbrook High School in the 1930s, when there were different rules for women and men. While men's basketball required five men to play the entire court, the women's basketball court was divided into three sections until 1938—and for many years after that, it was split into two sections—and women played either offense or defense but not both. We suspect that Mom played offense since her petite stature was ill suited for being a defender. In fact, Gary once recalled sitting up with friends late at night during his college days: "When we would talk about our families and they would ask me what my mom was like, I would say that she was short but sweet." Mom also played tennis, and she looked athletic.

Millie Homer, Mom's older sister by a few years, was slightly taller and also retained an athletic figure, which she kept trim by playing a lot more golf than my mother. Aunt Millie and her husband, Kip, had a membership at the country club. Mom, when she played golf later in life, went to local courses. Millie had the far more dominant personality. Millie and Kip also had two children, Fred, who was two years older than I, and Gail, who was six months younger. From my birth in 1941 until my graduation from high school in 1959, our families lived not much more than a foul shot away from each other.

When I was born, my first home was in an apartment on Long Island, in Lynbrook, New York, directly below the second-floor apartment occupied by my aunt and uncle. My mother's parents owned their own home a few blocks away. We moved to the nearby town of West Hempstead in 1951, when my folks and the Homers bought plots of land side by side. They had almost identical houses built at 366 and 372 School Street. Soon after our move to West Hempstead, my grandparents followed and built a one-story corner house around the block from our two homes. Mom and Dad remained at their School Street address until 1963, when Dad transferred to an office in Washington, DC. They then moved to nearby Adelphi, Maryland, across the border from Silver Springs and just down the road from the University of Maryland.

To us, as four children, it appeared that our parents all got along beautifully. And for the most part, that apparently was true. It certainly created a warm and nurturing environment to be raised, with two parents, an aunt, uncle, and two grandparents within walking distance of our home and a family who was together at important holidays and family events.

Cousin Gail offers a description of Mom's physical appearance and personality by contrasting her with Gail's mother, Millie: "When I think of your mom, it is always in contrast to my mom. My mom had dark hair; yours had blond. Mine had sharp edges; yours had soft edges. Mine was always on the go; yours was more relaxed. Millie was more fashion conscious; Aunt Rhoda was more sporty. Millie, more vocal and dominant; Rhoda, pretty easygoing. Both were pretty much under the thumb of Grandma too! I remember your mom and dad on the holiday trips to the Morse Farm in the Catskills and the walks we took and the easygoing, relaxed outdoor times that they were. And especially in the later years, I recall the continuing interest your mother took in us all. She was always inquiring and asking questions and probably knew more about our adult lives than my mom did. She continued to stay in touch even during that time, late in their lives, when she and my mother went without seeing or communicating with each other for close to a decade. And don't forget the power of the three together: my mother, your mother, and Grandma! I can still picture them all in Grandma's kitchen, drawing conclusions on one or another of us!"

Another contrast between our family and the Homers' is in the way we took vacations. Both families were what could be classified as middle class—neither wealthy nor close to poverty—but clearly the Homers had a better income than that provided by my dad's government job. Millie and Kip were good parents, and there was nothing to distinguish them from other conscientious parents of their day who occasionally made arrangements for their children so that they could take a holiday by themselves. But Mom and Dad expended what few resources they had for vacations on family trips. Often, cousins Gail and Fred would come with us. We usually went to the Morse Farm, a small, family operated bed-and-breakfast in the heart of the Catskill Mountains, in what was once known as the Borscht Belt, where comedians—mostly Jewish—performed at the resort hotels that dotted the area.

I recall with relish several aspects of these trips. One was the aroma of brewed coffee and the homemade baked goodies for breakfast. I truly believed that Chock Full of Nuts was, as sung in the ad, "that heavenly coffee." Of course, the fact that these trips were the only time I was allowed coffee and that I loaded each cup with five spoonfuls of sugar may have helped convince me that it was "heavenly." Also, I recall the small hill behind the farmhouse that seemed like a mountain to me at the time and the challenge of climbing the hill with our terrier mutt Buttons and the entire family along. And I remember romping, pushing and shoving, and tossing hay in the loft above the barn, with Gary, Gail, and Fred. Probably most of all, I recall the cheating scam at canasta that Fred and I concocted when he was about twelve, and I was around ten. If I said, "Fred, I think we should have two pancakes for breakfast tomorrow morning at nine," that meant I had a pair of nines. If he responded, "I'd rather have three pancakes at seven o'clock," then, of course, he had three sevens. It wasn't hard for the adults to see through our charade, but Mom never let on.

I realize now that Mom and Dad enjoyed vacations with us, and that's what made them vacations for them. Dad worked hard all week, and with more than a one-hour commute to New York City and back each morning and evening and a lot of fix-it work to do over the weekends, these three- or four-day family outings to the Morse Farm or occasional one-day trips to Bear Mountain—and a one-time trip to Florida with all of the Homers—were vacations for my parents as well as for us. But that was Mom. If we were happy, she was happy, and if she could watch us be happy, she was enjoying herself.

Trained as a bookkeeper, Rhoda Mesibov was a stay-at-home mom until I was in college and Gary was in high school. She then took a part-time job that she was recommended for by my Uncle Kip, who was a partner in an accounting firm in Hempstead. After Gary went off to college (Rutgers for a year and then Stanford), she changed to another bookkeeping job—this time at a cabana club in Lido Beach.

Mom was a traditional woman of the 1950s while I was growing up. She took responsibility for the cooking, the children, and the upkeep of the house, while Dad was the wage earner, the ultimate disciplinarian, Mr. Fix-It, and the final arbiter of important decisions. Her life was built around my brother and me, and it seemed that she was always in the house whenever we were—as well as when we weren't. She became an ardent Brooklyn Dodger fan when I, the oldest, decided to root for the Dodgers. Possibly I chose the Dodgers because my father was a Yankee fan or maybe because I was influenced by someone in the neighborhood—perhaps my older cousin Fred, with whom I played ball games of all sorts almost continuously as we were growing up.

In the 1950s, every Dodger game was on the radio, and most were on TV in the afternoon. Mom and I would watch the games together, and when the Dodgers were behind, it was my job to light a cigarette for her to provide the necessary luck the Dodgers would need to win the game. This seemed to almost always work. Whether it was because of a connection between the lighting of the cigarette and the ability of the Dodger players to hit or because the Dodgers had one of the best hitting teams of all time and were likely to score runs in the late innings with or without our help is for others to decide.

One of my saddest and simultaneously strongest memories occurred at 3:58 p.m. on Wednesday, October 3, 1951. I had arrived home from school a few minutes earlier and was still standing by the TV with my coat on as Ralph Branca came in to pitch for the Dodgers in the ninth inning, with Brooklyn leading 4–2. This was the day of "The Shot Heard 'round the World," when Bobby Thompson's three-run homer gave the Giants the pennant and a trip to the World Series. I stood stone-faced, mouth open in disbelief. Mom frequently would reminisce about the expression on my face but in the context of boasting of my persistence and using my loyalty to the Dodgers as an example.

It is curious that about the time Mom gave up smoking in 1957 (and would refrain from cigarettes for the rest of her life), the Dodgers began to encounter more difficulty winning and then moved to the West Coast. Mom praised her mother for having good instincts. Grandma Fanny had told Mom in the 1940s that cigarettes were no good for people—and this was a time when radio and newspaper ads spotlighted doctors singing the praises of tobacco. "Nine out of ten doctors recommend Camels," proclaimed the announcer during a commercial on Abbot and Costello's radio show. Mom respected her mother's instincts for what foods were healthy, and Grandma was often right. Ultimately, Mom listened to her mother and gave up smoking.

For Mother's Day or Mom's birthday at the end of June, Gary and I often gave her the gift of a visit to Ebbetts Field to see the Dodgers.

Mom encouraged our athletic pursuits, while never pushing us into activities—sports or otherwise. Gary played varsity baseball, football, and basketball, and she and Dad attended a lot of those games. Baseball was harder for them to attend because games were weekdays, but they came to those whenever they could, probably, Gary guesses, because it was his best sport, and he excelled as the team's catcher. And of course, Mom was an active member of the PTA and a supporter of our temple and Sunday school.

Gary recalls having a significant amount of quality time with both of our parents after he graduated from high school, when he lived with them for three summers shortly after they had moved to Maryland. "A main thing the three of us did together on the weekends when they moved to Adelphi was play golf. Mom always liked golf, and Dad got the okay to take it up from his doctor when they moved to Maryland, so we did that together many weekends, and they really enjoyed playing. We spent a lot of time together over those three summers because I did not have many friends down there, and neither did they when they first moved. We ate out a lot on the weekends and enjoyed each other's company. I spent the first summer working at the NY World's Fair, so I split time between New York and Maryland, but my last two summers there, I was working as a door-to-door salesman, selling a home-delivery food service run by the Jewel T Company—I think that was the name—which was a Midwest grocery store chain. And I was able to spend more time with Mom and Dad than had been possible since I had left home for college."

Interestingly, five years earlier, when I entertained thoughts of selling encyclopedias during the summer of 1960—a job that would pay no salary but a hefty commission for each sale—Mom cautioned me that it must be difficult to sell them. Mom's caution when I would discuss my sometimes risky ideas bothered me, in this case probably because I was much more nervous about committing to this job than my bravado would indicate. I was looking for reassurance, not doubt to add to the doubt I already had but wouldn't admit to. Gary recently speculated about the reason she embraced his decision to take a job as a salesman during his two full summers in Maryland: "You must have warmed her up to the idea of door-to-door selling because she was ecstatic when I got the job. Either it was your influence or she was just so happy to have me staying there with them during the summer."

Until he transferred to the Washington, DC office in 1963, Dad had put his law degree to work for nearly twenty years as an investigator for the Department of Agriculture out of an office in New York City. He would return home for a six-thirty dinner that Mom always had ready. This would consist of fish, hamburger, chicken, liver, or some kind of beef, a starch, a vegetable, and dessert—all of this preceded by an appetizer. The dessert was not always one for calorie- and cholesterol-conscious eaters. It was sometimes Jell-O or melon but often ice cream, cookies, or cake. Mom was not a frequent baker, but she did occasionally serve a homemade apple pie, my favorite dessert. This kind of diet was the norm in most homes those days, and our parents were not risk takers.

If I had one other complaint growing up, in addition to Mom's occasional cautious endorsement of some of my ideas, it was that she could be too quick to praise me for anything I did and to tell me how good I was. On the one hand, I did not react well to criticism, but on the other hand, knowing in advance that Mom would love anything I did—performance on the ball field, in a play, or on the snare drums, where it would be hard to find anyone with less talent—diminished the value of her kudos.

But this was Mom. As cousin Gail said recently, "I remember always thinking that she was the nicest person in the world, never having a mean thing to say about anyone. She was always happy, always smiling. I don't remember ever seeing her upset. In her later years, when she and Ed were in Florida, I remember looking forward to our annual trip to see my parents because Aunt Rhoda always smiled, and she was always so glad to see me."

Another of Gary's recollections of Mom is described in something he said to a colleague that he is sure he learned from our mother. In a note that began, "There is never a dull moment," the colleague had related that she had a man over to talk about problems with her deck. He said that there was no immediate crisis, but it needed some work, and they should start planning that soon. According to Gary, "I wrote back and said I agreed that there is always something, but at least there is no immediate danger. Then I thought about what I wrote to her and realized that is exactly what Mom would say. She often talked about what a hassle things were and dwelled on that a bit, but never for too long because she then quickly moved to the bright side of the situation." Mom's glass was definitely filled halfway all the time.

Recently I asked each of her five grandchildren, along with Susan, Laurie, Gary, and Gail, to summarize who my mother was in one word or phrase. Without seeing each other's responses, Marli and Susan each cited the same characteristic: *gentle*. Marli's recollection was: "If I were able to sum up who Grandma was in one word or phrase, it would be *gentle*. She was always smiling, always considerate, and gentle toward the people around her."

Susan reminisces about her mother-in-law:
I remember being on the golf course with her, and she was the most relaxed golf player! She taught me that it wasn't important what the score was: if the shot was bad, take another one; if you don't like the lie, move the ball. We aren't professionals; we're just enjoying ourselves!

Darren reminisces about his grandmother:
The quality I admired most in her was her consistent, unshakable, friendly disposition.

Mom's report card, freshman
year at Lynbrook High School.

Lynbrook Girls Win at Nets, 3-2

Down Freeport in Close Contest at Marion Street Courts

Rhoda Rubenstein's victory over Helen Wright in the second singles match gave the Lynbrook high school girls tennis team a 3-2 win over the Freeport girls net team in a closely fought engagement at the Marion street courts, Lynbrook yesterday afternoon.

Miss Rubenstein's victory over Miss Wright was scored in straight sets, but the first one was extended to 22 games, and the second to 13 before a decision was reached.

Write-up in local paper as Mom won her tennis match.

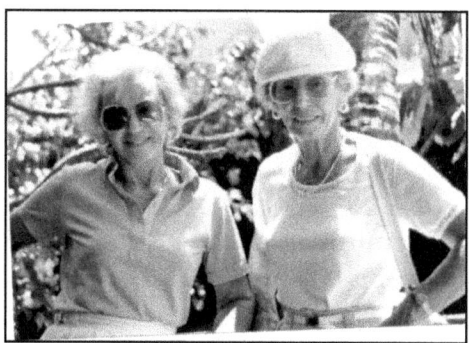

Sisters Millie and Rhoda several years before Mom's Alzheimer's began to reveal itself.

Chapter 4

A Father-and-Son Relationship

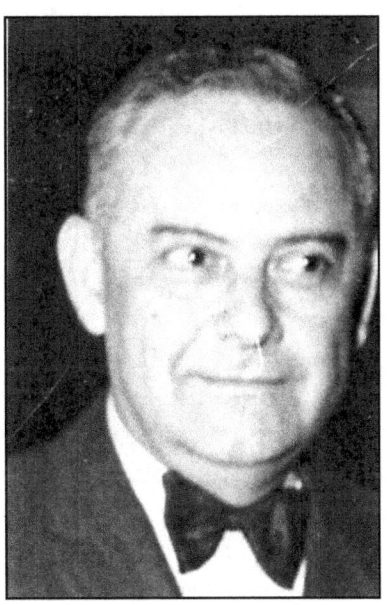

Harold Mesibov, Mom's first husband.

The flight back to New York for me was a time for reflection. I thought about Ed lying in the hospital about to die, and I thought of the time I learned of my first father's death.

Appreciating Mom Through the Lens of Alzheimer's

That Saturday I was on the ball field of Camp Regis, a summer camp in the Adirondack Mountains in upstate New York, when the phone call came from my mother: "Dad died this morning." I drove the seven hours to West Hempstead for the funeral. Mom was devastated and said she didn't know how she could go on living. I'm sure she was not suicidal, but she could not find any hope looking to the future. I was twenty-five and single, living in my insulated world in which I had experienced only one death of someone close, that of my grandfather, the year before. I was frustrated and hurt that I couldn't convince Mom that her children should be enough to sustain her will to live.

How did I react to losing my father? There was respect, admiration, love, and a certain distance. I'm not sure I can say that I felt close to him. Just as Mom was the stereotypical mother of the 1940s and '50s, so was Dad the stereotypical good father of that era. He was 100 percent a family man. He was a product of growing up through the Depression. After seeing his father lose everything in the 1929 stock market crash, he was fiscally conservative and had an excellent work ethic and a strong sense of what was right and wrong.

My dad loved me very much, but our communications were superficial, and I never viewed him as someone to confide in. I was always excited when he and Mom came to visit me at camp twice each summer, and I couldn't wait for them to observe me playing softball or see me in the lead role in the camp play, which I often had. One of my parents was almost always at my little league games, and I recall the one time neither could make it, and Grandpa came instead. Perhaps the reason my memory of that day is so vivid is because I made the error that cost us the game, and Grandpa consoled me on the ride home. Mom came right into my room when she got home, and she did all she could to let me know that I would live to play another game.

Now that I am a parent, I realize even more how much my parents sacrificed—financially and otherwise—to send me to camp, take vacations with the whole family, and see that Gary and I had whatever it was possible for our family to afford. I recognize that Dad's life and my mother's revolved around what Gary and I needed and wanted.

I think the difference between good fathers in that era and today is that fathers then assumed the role of providers, while fathers today, including myself I hope, try to connect more with their children as well as to provide for them.

The effect of Dad's sudden passing was probably more long term than immediate for me. Knowing that my parents would always be there for me was a source of security. For instance, I never had to ask for money once they had paid my way through college, but the knowledge that Dad and Mom would never let me starve or go without shelter enabled me to live on the brink of financial insolvency without worrying about it. I wasn't reliant on my father, and that's why I think the impact of his passing was more long-term than at the moment I heard the news. During our weekly phone conversations, Mom would tell me what Dad was doing, and she'd end with "Dad sends his love." From the time I left home to go to college and after I graduated but remained in the Boston area for several years, I'd travel to visit them at least once a year. They'd come to Boston to celebrate my birthday, for special events, or if we hadn't seen each other in a while. But I was still "finding" myself, and while I knew that Dad would be there for me in a crisis, I wasn't personally secure enough to rely on him for advice. Had he lived longer, I'm sure we would have spent more time together in meaningful conversation, on vacations, and with more frequent visits, as happened with my mother after I married, had children of my own, and matured to where I was as interested in my parents' lives as I assumed they would be in mine.

When I graduated from Boston University, I spent a year in a futile attempt to raise funds for the purchase of an overnight summer camp, and I supported myself—barely—by working as a cashier at the Star Market in Brookline, a suburb of Boston. I had the impression that my dad disapproved and would have preferred that I had gone straight from college into a more traditional occupation with an annual salary.

Yet years after his passing, Mom assured me that Dad always had confidence that I would land on my feet. She would quote him, saying, "Donnie has a good head on his shoulders; Donnie will do all right." This has always meant a lot to me. I wish I had known it at the time, and that's why I frequently try to find ways to let my children know how proud and supportive I am of them as each pursues dramatically different, but equally worthwhile, pathways toward success, happiness, and service to others.

Four days after Dad's death, I was back at Camp Regis, glad that Gary would be with my mother for the summer and confident that my assurances that I would be available at the drop of a hat would be sufficient to reassure her. Yet at the advanced level of maturity that twenty-five years of living had afforded me (self-absorbed might be a more nearly accurate description), I couldn't understand how she wasn't focused on the important role that she would have to play in the lives of my brother and me and, eventually, our families. I guess if I thought about it, I just assumed that death was something you grieved for a while, and then you put it behind you and continued moving forward with your life. The truth is probably that I didn't think about it except how it would affect me. Being athletic director at summer camp was a very important part of my life, probably too important for me to be able to put it in perspective in the light of my dad's death. Taking a few days off was one thing; missing some of the events I had planned and was expected to supervise was another. On one level I was shaken, and I understood that my mother would be deeply affected. On another level, I was too involved with my personal goals to have given deep thought to how her life would change.

At the time of Dad's death in July, I had been hired to work as a weekly newspaper editor in Concord, Massachusetts, to begin as soon as my summer camp job ended in September. Gary was continuing his education en route to joining the faculty at the University of North Carolina in 1974, where he rapidly became a pioneer in the field of autism and a world-recognized authority on the subject. He and the director of his department coauthored ten books on the topic of autism before 1980.

Several months after Dad died, Mom moved back to West Hempstead, where she took an upstairs bedroom in the home of my aunt and uncle. Two rooms had been vacated by my cousins, Gail and Fred, who were then grown and on their own. My grandmother, widowed a year and a half earlier in February 1965, lived in an extension built especially for her off the kitchen.

A few years later, Mom met Ed Meister, a widower with two grown children, who was living in the neighboring town of Hempstead and practicing medicine in nearby Franklin Square. They were married May 14, 1971 and bought a one-story house with a guest room and master bedroom in Royal Palm Beach, Florida. Initially this was a winter retreat as Ed gradually reduced his workload, and it was a place for all four of their children to visit and bring their families. It finally became their year-round home a few years later as Ed divested himself completely of his Franklin Square practice.

Until Mom's Alzheimer's and Ed's fall in the shower, they were blessed with remarkably good health. They continued their automobile treks up north to visit both Mesibov families every summer until the late 1990s, when, as he passed the age of ninety, Ed became reluctant to travel far from home—more for fear of a medical problem occurring while he was away than from the reality of any actual concern. Ed's hospitalization was his first significant physical setback since he and Mom were wed. And now it was almost thirty years since their wedding, and Larry was on the phone calling to say that Ed could go at any time. He did, in fact, pass the next day. Having had a month to anticipate the loss of Ed, Susan and I had decided, and Gary concurred, that the only viable alternative for our mother was to bring her to Potsdam, where at least one of the four of us was almost always in the house. Susan taught special education full time, but she was home by four o'clock on most days. I worked from home as an educational consultant, and my meetings were almost always late afternoon or at night. While Marli and Raina had busy after-school schedules, often one or the other was home soon after the end of the school day.

By contrast, both of our nephews, Brian and Todd, were out of the nest and on their way to becoming successful attorneys, and Gary and Laurie were out of their house most days. Laurie, an attorney, worked for the university in Chapel Hill, and Gary's work included travel around the world, helping communities and organizations set up their own autism programs. When we had been looking for a retirement home for Mom and Ed, the Chapel Hill area would have been ideal because Laurie and Gary would have been able to visit frequently and could have been available at a moment's notice. However, with the situation changed and our sense that Mom would benefit from having family around all the time, we agreed that Susan, Marli, Raina, and I were in the best position to provide what Mom needed, and Darren was able to make frequent visits from Arizona to help out.

Sue and I decided that Raina would travel with me to Florida for Ed's funeral and then bring Mom back with us, while she and Marli would stay in Potsdam and tend to the myriad details involved in preparing for a full-time guest who would need special attention. We also agreed to ask Alice if she would be willing to come to Potsdam for a short time to help transition Mom to a local caregiver.

Gary reminisces about his mother:
The time I remember most being with Mom was when the family came to my graduation at Stanford in 1967. I think it was the first big trip she took after Dad died the previous summer and the first time I saw her really happy since then. It made me feel good that she seemed ready to move on.

Todd reminisces about his grandmother:
I don't know what I would have said when I was growing up, but now I'm impressed with how tough she was.

Chapter 5

Mom Moves to Potsdam

Ed passed away on Thursday, September 28, 2000. Three days later Gary's and Laurie's first grandchild, Anna, was born to their oldest son Brian and their daughter-in-law Sally. The proximity of the time of death of an older person and the entry into the world of a baby in the same family is eerily similar to what happened to us two days after Marli was born. We had to inform Susan while she lay in her hospital bed with Marli in her arms that her Uncle Stanley, to whom she was close, had passed away from heart failure.

In Jewish tradition, Ed's funeral should have been the next day, but for various reasons it could not be held until the following Monday. With my encouragement, Gary returned to North Carolina on Sunday, the day before Ed's funeral. Everything was under control, and it was clear that we would need Gary to return—probably a few times—to attend to details such as meetings with attorneys, bankers, or brokers and going through everything in their now-vacated apartment. Sunday afternoon the five of us—Raina, Larry, Dee, Mom, and I—traveled to the funeral home. Mom, Raina, and I were left alone to view the body. Mom didn't cry, either during the viewing or at any time during or after the funeral. But she seemed very much aware of what was happening. She didn't seem moved at any time during the funeral rites. All afternoon she kept commenting on how peaceful Ed looked. Raina broke down and sobbed after being at the viewing for a while—it was a healthy experience for her—and she cried again at the funeral.

Unfortunately their regular rabbi was out of town, but his alternate did a wonderful job. He was sensitive and said all the right things Sunday evening when he came to the house to get background information for Monday's funeral. He conducted a beautiful service. There were twenty-one people at graveside and about that at the reception following, which was held in the back of the dining hall at The Classic.

Mom was pretty good at the funeral and reception. Her friend Rae was there and was quite alert and seemingly healthy. It was good to see her. Rae was so much like Mom, always asking questions, always showing a genuine interest in what we were doing and what we had to say. Rae and Lenny Horowitz had been the closest friends of my mother and father since the early 1950s. For a couple of summers, they sent their son, Alan, to Camp Balfour, the eight-week overnight summer camp in the Adirondacks that I lived for from the age of seven until I was a counselor at the age of twenty-two, in 1963. Gary began at a similar age. Rae, Lenny, Mom, and Dad would travel ten hours by car for parent-visiting weekends, and often they would turn them into longer vacations.

After Dad passed away, Ed and my mother resumed the close relationship when Rae and Lenny moved to Florida, only a few miles from their Royal Palm Beach home. Lenny lost his battle with Alzheimer's about a year before Ed's passing. As we said goodbye at the reception, I promised Rae—as well as Mom's friend, Edna, and anyone else there for Mom—that we would bring Mom to visit when we came back to clear out her things. This promise, it turned out, was not one that I was able to keep.

The more time I spent with Mom, the more evidence I saw of her memory loss, notwithstanding the memory pills she had apparently been taking for at least four months. Mom often brought up Ed's name as if we had just left him or were about to see him, and each time I reminded her he had recently died. She accepted my reminders as matter-of-factly as if I had asked her to pass the salt. There was no emotion as we discussed Ed. She listened to my explanation of his death, and shortly after she repeated, "I need to get home to make Ed some dinner." Alzheimer's was insulating Mom from the grief she had experienced when Dad passed away.

During our family visit to Florida at the end of August, and again when Raina and I went down in late September for the funeral, we had quite a few dinners with Aunt Millie and her new husband, Mel. They lived in Boynton Beach, less than a half hour from the hospital, so we saw them several times during our brief trips to Florida after Ed's fall. Millie had enjoyed sixty years of marriage to Kip. After he passed away September 22, 1996, following several severe strokes and a long stay in a nursing home, she married Mel, a widower also living in Florida. They were good company for each other, and Mel's calm disposition was a tonic for Millie who can be impulsive at times. Before he headed back to Chapel Hill on Sunday, the day before the funeral, Gary joined us at several of these restaurant meals, as did Larry and Dee.

At one dinner, Aunt Millie kept asking what our plans were, and her face revealed her disapproval each time I said that we were taking Mom up north with us. Aunt Millie then continued to refer to "the plan" she had for Mom and the many friends Mom had who would keep her busy in Florida. She meant well, but all I could think of was how few people were still willing to spend any time with Mom. Even if Aunt Millie and a few others joined her for dinner once or twice a week, how would Mom occupy her time the rest of the week? Besides, Aunt Millie didn't understand—or hadn't accepted—that Mom needed someone with her almost all the time due to the deterioration already evident in her memory and the loss of skills that were dependent on her memory, such as driving.

Midafternoon the day following the funeral, Aunt Millie and Mel said good-bye. Mel told me, out of Millie's hearing, how much he admired the way Gary and I took charge of things and how well he felt I had handled "both ladies" with patience during the meal the night before.

I heaved a sigh of relief when Raina, Mom, Alice, and I were on the plane. We had pairs of seats, one pair in front of the other. My thought had been that Alice would sit with Mom, and Raina and I would sit together, but Raina wanted to sit next to Mom, and I thought that was great. About a quarter of the time, Raina kept Mom busy by discussing her Build-A-Bear animals. She had created one in Vermont on a family vacation a year or two before, and when Gary had taken her for a few hours while we were visiting Ed in the hospital, they had returned with another from a store that he had located near West Palm Beach. The other three-fourths of the time Raina patiently answered Mom's "Where are we going?" questions: "Grandma, we'll be in Atlanta at 8:50 p.m.; we'll leave at 9:50; we'll be in Syracuse at midnight; we'll stay in a Best Western; and we'll drive to Potsdam tomorrow morning."

When I heard Mom ask about our itinerary a fourth time, I hastily wrote on a piece of paper, "Arrive Atlanta, 9 pm, depart at 10 pm, arrive Syracuse midnight," and I handed it to her. The next time she asked Raina when we would arrive, Raina said, "We'll be in Atlanta at 8:50." Mom looked at her paper and said, "But it says 9 pm." Raina responded, "Dad was just being approximate on the paper; we'll actually be there at 8:50 and leave at 9:50." Mom kept looking at the paper and telling Raina what was written on it. Finally, Raina, after trying in vain to convince Mom that the times on the paper were approximate, asked me for a pen and changed them. "There, Grandma, it says on the paper that we are arriving at 8:50, and that's when we will arrive."

When we left Atlanta, at 9:50, Raina again asked to sit next to Grandma. She occupied her and kept her comfortable on the second flight.

Darren reminisces about his grandmother:
Being with Grandma made me feel relaxed and friendly.

Raina reminisces about her grandmother:
Being with Grandma made me feel safe, loved.

Mom Moves to Potsdam

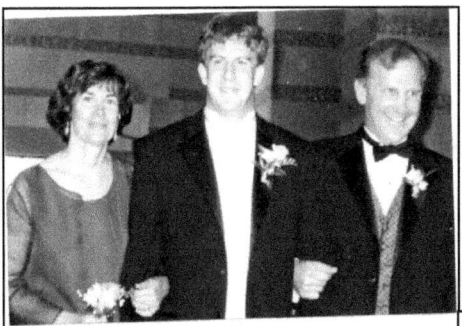

Mom's son Gary with his wife, Laurie, and their younger son, Todd, at his wedding to Katie, May 26, 2001.

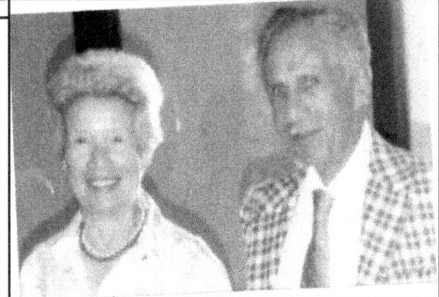

Rae and Lenny Horowitz, Mom's closest friends during both of her marriages.

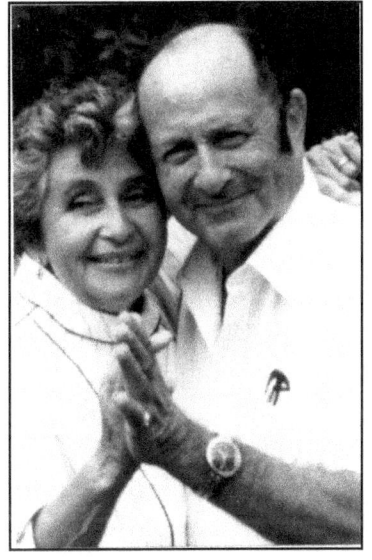

Susan's Aunt Gloria and Uncle Stanley. He passed away two days after Marli's birth. Uncle Stanley was a pilot. In addition to crop dusting he often flew celebrities to concert dates; among the most famous was Dionne Warwick. Uncle Stanley often spoke of how he turned down an offer by one of his passengers to invest in a show that was about to be produced on Broadway. He felt that it was too ethnic to be appreciated by a wide enough audience to be successful. The show was *Fiddler on the Roof*.

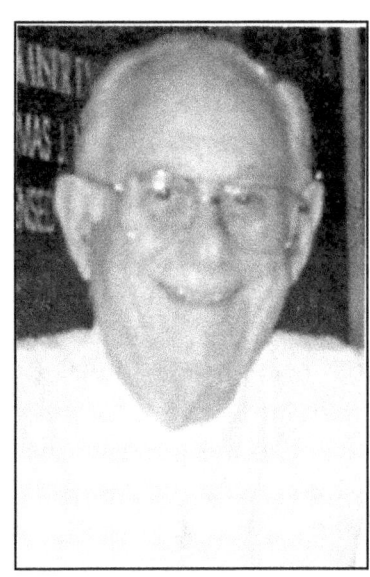

Mom's sister, Millie, married Mel Hershenson (pictured) late in life, after the passing of Uncle Kip.

Chapter 6

Laughter and Pathos

Friday, October 6

We arrived in Syracuse after midnight and stayed in the Airport Best Western. This morning we drove two and a half hours to our home in Potsdam and immediately took Mom for a visit with Dr. Kay. He has been our family physician since Marli's birth in 1985, when a friend recommended him to be our pediatrician. He appears to be about fifty, with graying hair, medium build, and medium height.

Dr. Kay told us that he had a family member with Alzheimer's, and he inspired our confidence both in the way he treated Mom and in the way he described the characteristics of Alzheimer's and how they differed from other forms of dementia. "Some memory loss is inevitable as we age, but Alzheimer's is much more extreme." Dr. Kay's strength, in addition to an excellent diagnostic ability, is his bedside manner. No matter how many patients he has waiting, he conveys the impression that you can have as much time as you need. He spoke conversationally with Mom as he asked her to identify the state she had lived in, the state she is in now, her country, and the year of her birth. She did pretty well with her responses and was particularly impressive counting backward from a hundred and getting into the 80s. I tried to count backward with her silently and had a little difficulty, but then again, Mom was a bookkeeper.

Saturday, October 7

I received an e-mail that my cousin Gail sent from her home in England: "Thank you for your message. This is all very sad, and it is harder as we are all so far away from one another. I would have very much liked to have come to Ed's funeral to be with you all and say good-bye to Ed, whom we liked and respected enormously. Your mom sounded very confused when I spoke to her but also so like her kind self. My mother is also confused, but I hadn't quite taken aboard the extent to which you have noticed. What are the memory pills? Do they know about them? I will suggest them for my mother. Do they prevent deterioration? I also notice that my mother gets much worse when she gets stressed, and probably that is the same with your mother. How are you all managing now? I'm sorry this is such a difficult time. I'll call later today. Love to all."

A book Gary recommended, *The 36-Hour Day*, arrived in the mail. We placed it in a basket, where Sue and I could both start reading whenever the opportunities arose. It turned out to be extremely helpful.

Gail called in the afternoon (late night for Londoners); however, before I handed the phone to Mom, Gail asked whether she had more difficulty remembering things when she was stressed. I indicated that was true, and that she also was far less mentally sharp in general when she was tired. Gary had noticed that if he wanted to communicate something important to Mom, the morning was usually a better time. We also believe that Mom is sharper right after she's taken her twice-daily pills. The memory pills are relatively new on the market, a prescription medication called Exelon, and they really do seem to help a lot.

I shared some stories with Gail about our recent times in Florida with her mother and mine: "Gail, being with our mothers was not without its lighter moments. When we were down in August and Ed had just entered the hospital, it was clear that we had to prevent Mom from driving. With Ed in the car, she was okay, but without him, as he had told us, 'She'd never find her way home.' So we hid the keys. She kept looking for them and asking 'Anyone seen my keys?' I kept putting her off, saying, 'We'll find them later, Mom.'

"Gary went down a week later and told me that somehow Mom decided that your mother had the keys. So every time your mother would come over, Mom would ask 'Did you find my keys, Millie?' Your mother became convinced that she must have the keys. Gary said that periodically Aunt Millie would come over and have a different key, and she would ask 'Is this it?'

"Mom stopped her obsession with the keys, but even this past week, on a few occasions, she has said, 'You know I loaned the keys to the car to Millie, and she can't find them.'

"While in Florida between the time of the funeral and our return to Potsdam a few days later, there were some moments with your mother and mine that were both sad because of the gradual deterioration that is taking place in both of their minds and also comical because their interactions were so typical, in many ways, of their personalities.

"Dinner at a restaurant is a slow process with my mother, as you know. It can take her ten minutes to decide on a menu item. The other night, your mother and Mel joined us again for dinner. Your mother had begun lobbying loudly with me the previous night for a third straight dinner at Boston Chicken, but Dee and Larry helped me dissuade her, using the argument that Raina wanted something different, which she did. We all went to Applebee's over your mother's resigned, 'Well, only for you, Raina.'

"Our mothers quickly agreed to split a chicken salad plate (after Aunt Millie lamented that she had received only three scrawny pieces of chicken with her salad the last time she had been to Applebee's). As the rest of us took our time deciding, I thought that at least your mother's presence had helped my mother make a quick decision on the dinner order.

"The waiter came and took my order, then Raina's, then Mel's, then Larry's, and then Dee's. Then he looked toward your mother and mine. They decided they really didn't want the salad they had decided on. 'I only got three pieces of chicken the last time I ordered it,' your mother repeated. 'Then let's get something else,' my mom chimed in.

"Now we were back to square one and had wasted all the time we had been sitting waiting for the server to come, thinking that they knew what they wanted. My mother (for at least the sixth time) said, 'What are you having, Donnie?'

"'The fajita, Mom,' I answered, holding up a picture of the special on the menu.

"'What's a fajita?' Once again I responded. Ten minutes and several menu items later, my mom asked 'What are you having, Donnie?'

"'The fajita, Mom. Here's a picture of it.'

"'I think I'll have that too. Millie, what are you going to have?'

"'Maybe I'll have that too. Last time I had the chicken salad and they only brought me three pieces of chicken.'

"I thought the fajita was a good choice for my mother since I knew she'd like the chicken and figured she could pick and choose from the items that come with it. When the food came, the fajita plates were piled high with chicken, peppers, lettuce, tomato, onions, and sauces. Your mother took one look at it and exclaimed, 'My God, we should have gotten one order for the two of us—we'll never finish this.' I couldn't resist. 'At least, Aunt Millie,' I said, 'you should have plenty of chicken.' Your mother finished everything on her plate.

"On a more serious note, during our dinners together your mother conversed intelligently, but while it was hard to be certain, I saw evidence of what I thought were the beginning stages of Alzheimer's. Your mother appeared to be where my mom was several years ago.

"When she kept pushing to have Mom remain in Florida, I tried to avoid arguing with her, but I made it clear that the decision had been made and was not up for negotiation. Mom was returning with Raina and me; Alice would accompany us on the trip north."

As I recounted the stories of our mothers' interactions, Gail had difficulty controlling her laughter and finally commented: "What is so amazing is that despite the memory loss, the basic personality issues remain! Need I say more? But whatever my mother forgets, will she *ever* forget Boston Chicken? Your mom seems to be settling down nicely. She's very lucky to have you all. A friend of mine's mom has Alzheimer's, and she has taken to writing down answers to questions that she repeatedly asks so that her mother can read the sheet to reassure herself. It sounds like you have a good doctor. This week I am out of the office until Friday, but I will try to ring again to say hello next weekend. It's so good to talk with you. Let me talk with your mother."

Sunday, October 8

Our two-story Northern New York home is in the rural town of Potsdam, less than forty minutes from the Canadian border. It rests on four and a half acres of land and is identified by local people as "the home set way back from the road and covered with flower gardens." There is a finished basement, which includes a large office that Susan and I share, an equally large recreation room that was designed for our children to use, and a separate narrow area for storage, a washing machine, and a dryer. This, in effect, gives us living space on three floors.

On the top floor is our master bedroom at the opposite end of a narrow hallway, eighteen feet from the large guest room that became Mom's when we returned from Florida. As you climb the stairs toward this top floor, if you make an immediate left, it is two steps to enter the master bedroom. If you turn right, you pass Marli's room on the right, a full bathroom on the left, and then Raina's bedroom on the left. If you don't turn to enter Raina's room, you will walk straight ahead into Mom's room. The main floor has a dining room, living room, family room and adjacent kitchen, a den, and a half bathroom. The den and the half bathroom are directly across a narrow hallway from each other.

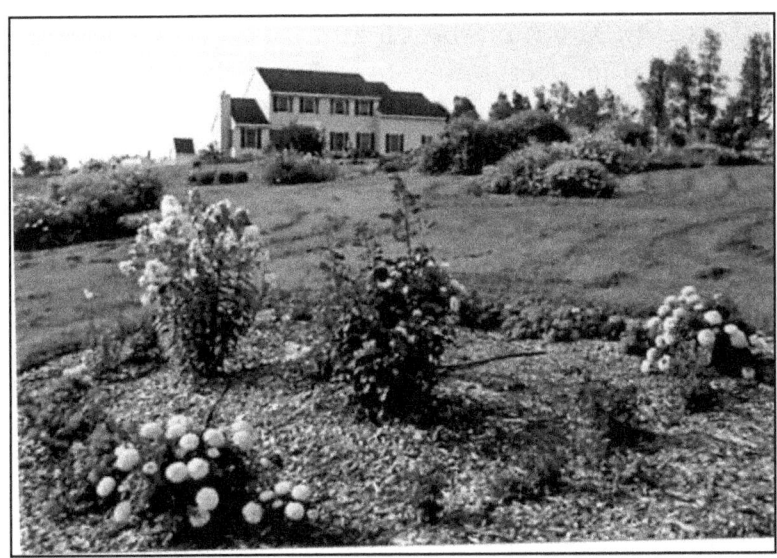

Our home in Potsdam, New York, on four and a half acres of property.

Early this morning, Sue found Mom wandering the upstairs hallway and into our bedroom. When she spotted Sue, Mom asked, "Where's the bathroom?" Sue told Mom she could use the bathroom in our master bedroom or the one she just passed halfway down the hallway. Mom headed for our bathroom, turned, and wanted to know, "How come I don't have a bathroom in my room? I guess I chose the wrong room."

Sue speculates that Mom thinks she is in a hotel.

Shortly afterward, I walked upstairs to the main floor, one flight up from my home office in the basement, and I saw Mom and Alice reading as Mom waited for the thirty minutes to pass from the time she took her pill until she could have breakfast. "I'll be back in a few minutes to join you for breakfast, Mom," I said.

"Where are you going?" she asked.

"Do I *have* to tell you?" I asked jokingly.

"Yes," she smiled.

"Okay, I'm going to the bathroom."

"Why this one?" she asked, referring to the main floor lavatory.

"Actually, Mom, maybe I'll go across the street to use the neighbor's; it's the nicest one in town."

"Good idea," she said, smiling and seeming to understand that I was teasing, although I doubt she understood the nature of the tease.

Alice and Mom set up a pill organizer for the week. It will prove to be a big help. Also, we posted a large calendar in her room and will cross off each day as it passes so she can identify the date by noticing the first date that doesn't have a mark through it. This also will enable her to identify the day of the week on the pill organizer that is appropriate.

Mom had it rough at times today in terms of disorientation and inability to sit still or stay with any one thing too long. She had many questions about where she is, at times being sure she is on Long Island, and she frequently mixed up her two marriages or completely forgot some of her personal history.

The girls each put a sign on their door with their name on it, and they put a sign up for their grandmother, saying, "Mom's Room." This is a variation on a suggestion by the doctor. I had told Marli and Raina that Dr. Kay had said that they really needed to put ribbon or yarn across all doors except Mom's and use a totally different symbol (such as the "Mom's Room" sign) over Mom's door. She needs to be able to identify, at a quick glance at night, which room is hers and which rooms aren't.

Mom's mood continues to be delightful. I am amazed at how friendly and cooperative she remains with everyone she meets, whether she has known them in the past or they are a neighbor stopping by to drop something off, introduced to her for the first time. As I read the *The 36-Hour Day*, I realize how lucky we are. The author speaks of how people react differently to Alzheimer's: some are pleasant and delightful, like Mom, while some become moody, depressed, and unpleasant to be with. Even when their personalities are normally pleasant, some people become mean-spirited with this disease. We are so fortunate that her true personality shines through despite the disease; if anything, it is becoming magnified through this process.

Mom also seems to be having an easier time accepting her frequent state of confusion as her confidence grows in Gary or me always being right by her side. She had said to me in Florida, "A lot of people mean well, but you and Gary are the only ones I can rely on. I need you." Consistent with this, she accepts any suggestion I make or explanation I give, without challenge. She is also starting to accept Sue, the children, and Alice in the same vein, but it is a transference from Gary and me. If Gary or I put her in a situation, she seems to trust it and go with it. As she gets to know the people closest to us and sees that we respect and trust them, so does she.

This afternoon we survived a call from Aunt Millie, who, after quizzing me on Mom's status, asked to speak with her! I listened in so that I could help Mom understand what Millie was saying, and I heard Millie encouraging Mom to fly to Florida. "Come on back to Boynton Beach so we can take care of you, Rhoda," I heard Millie say. Fortunately, Mom thinks Millie is still living on Long Island, and she cannot understand why Millie wants her to fly to Florida.

I described this conversation to Gary over the phone a few minutes after Aunt Millie hung up, and I said, "Aunt Millie is urging Mom to come and stay at her house with her and Mel. I think the relevant question would be: after two days, when Aunt Millie can no longer handle having Mom in the house, what would she propose next?" Gary's immediate response was, "Are you sure it would take two days to reach this point?"

Mom was excited that we were going to temple this evening to celebrate Kol Nidre, the start of Yom Kippur, the Day of Atonement. She seemed to really look forward to it. Just as the rabbi was so much solace to her at the funeral in Florida, I think that any time spent in religious observance is important to her because it is among the few staples she has had in her life that she can still have—and she seems to cling to these even more now as so much around her becomes fuzzier. It's not that Gary and I were brought up in a super religious environment. Our family celebrated the High Holy Days, we went to Sunday school, and the family occasionally went to Friday night services. In fact, Fred and I used to get through the rabbi's sermons by counting the number of words he would use that began with a particular letter of the alphabet. At the end of a sermon, neither of us could recall a single thing he had said, but we could tell you that he had begun 117 words with the letter *D*. While my family practiced Reform Judaism, Sue's family belonged to an Orthodox Synagogue in Long Beach, New York. In fact, the separation of men and women in an Orthodox temple presents a paradox that I occasionally kid Susan about since it pits a sexist tradition against the feminist beliefs Susan marched for in the 1960s. However, she is far from the only person to allow religious tradition to coexist with current, contradictory beliefs.

Mom wanted to call Gary, so we placed the call. Gary wasn't home, but Mom had a conversation with Laurie. We went to temple, and Mom was attentive. She sat calmly for almost two hours. However when we returned home at eight o'clock, she complained of a stomachache and wanted to take medicine; we gave her Maalox. She also complained of a headache.

Monday, October 9

Last Friday night we gave Mom her sleeping pill at ten o'clock, but it was eleven thirty before she finished her round trips to the bathroom to get ready for bed. Saturday night we gave her the pill at eight o'clock and didn't start trying to move her to bed until nine thirty. She was asleep by ten and slept through. So last night we again began the process at eight o'clock. Getting Mom into bed, however, was another story. It often takes her about an hour to finish revising items in the bathroom and searching drawers. But at least last night, once she got into bed, she slept through. This morning I called Gary and described this problem. He said, "Alice had a big problem with this throughout the time of Ed's hospitalization. There must be some strategies for dealing with this, so perhaps we can discuss it this weekend when we will be in Florida together."

Our plan is for me to take Mom with me so that Gary can see her and so that we can all go through her apartment at The Classic, clear things out, and decide who should take what and what should be sold, discarded, or given away. It will also be the time that I can accompany Alice back to Florida. Ginny, a local caregiver highly recommended by a friend of Sue's, starts work today so that it will allow us five days to transition from Alice to Ginny as Mom's daytime caregiver.

Laurie agreed to look over the lease agreement with The Classic—which committed Mom and Ed to at least eighteen more months—so that she can advise us if we have the right to cancel the lease sooner than its expiration date. If Laurie is able to offer an opinion before next weekend, we may seek a meeting with a representative of The Classic. I asked Gary to see if Laurie had a copy of the agreement because, if not, I will fax it to her. I have read it over, and based on my twenty-three years of prior experience as a labor-relations specialist for the teachers' union, the contract seems firm on the two-year obligation that began the previous May. This would mean we'd be paying for another eighteen months with no one in the apartment. However, the last page summarizes penalties for early departure—a couple of months of rent, which could be interpreted to allow for early departure as long as you pay the penalties.

I started an agenda of items for Gary and me to address when we meet in Florida, and I put the lease at the top of the list. The agenda is a work in progress:

1. The lease with The Classic
2. Financial handling—all aspects, how many accounts, what do we charge to Mom's accounts, etc.
3. Legal questions
4. Accounting questions
5. Ultimate home for Mom?
6. Questions for Larry
7. Questions for doctor
8. Disposition of their car
9. Sleeping pills and sleep habits

This morning when Mom awakened, she continued to emphasize that something isn't right, that she just doesn't feel that good, and "What's wrong with me?" A few tears escaped my eyes as I wondered: are these just brief periods of reality that break through her inability to think straight, or is she in frequent agony, able to understand that something terrible is happening to her mind?

By ten thirty she seemed much better, and we went to temple for Yom Kippur morning services. Again she sat through more than two hours of services, stayed on the appropriate page, and read well whenever she could locate the place. Once again she really seemed to take comfort in going to temple and being in that environment. The services ended shortly after one o'clock. We went home, and she napped for over ninety minutes (getting up for trips to the bathroom three times, but sleeping soundly in between).

On Yom Kippur it is Jewish tradition not to eat or drink anything from sundown one day to sundown the next. We broke this fast downstairs at the temple after a two-hour service this evening, and Mom probably ate more at this meal than at any time I have been with her, even though she hadn't fasted the previous twenty-four hours with the rest of us. A retired professor named Dorothy (a nice person, but one who can chat at length without giving a listener a chance to interact) sat across from Mom and was wearing a "Hillary for Senate" campaign button. During dessert, while others at the table, including Sue, had gone for coffee or had left the table to seek out other friends, Dorothy leaned toward Mom and started espousing her political and philosophical views. Dorothy spoke continuously and uninterrupted for at least ten minutes until Mom moved her head in Dorothy's direction, focused on the campaign button on Dorothy's blouse, and asked, "Where are you from, Hillary?"

We arrived home about eight thirty, and Mom tried calling Gary; then Alice gave Mom her pill. Mom filled a glass with water and went to put it in the crowded refrigerator. Alice, trying to be helpful, said, "Rhoda, don't put that glass in the refrigerator, you can get fresh water in the morning." But Sue smiled and told Alice, "It's her ritual, Alice. When Ed was alive, they would put two glasses in the refrigerator to get cold overnight or to be there for a late-night drink before bedtime."

Alice has been terrific, and Sue frequently comments about it, although Sue was skeptical when I first proposed bringing Alice back here for a few weeks. Now Sue has gone from wondering why we wanted to bring Alice here to asking Alice, "What will it take to keep you here?" In fact when I called Sue from Florida a week ago and urged bringing Alice with us as Dee and Larry had suggested, she initially said, "Even Raina asked what we need Alice for." I thought about that, and then in a later conversation, I suggested that Raina was so proud of how well she had cared for Grandma in Florida that she figured she could handle it without Alice in Potsdam. I think that was Raina's reference point. I explained to Raina that we needed Alice for the times Raina would be in school or doing homework. As Alice got up to collect our plates from the table, Sue said to her, "We're getting spoiled. What will we do after you leave?"

In contrast to Sue's changed opinion, Raina has gone from being Alice's playmate in Florida to being ready for her to leave—to the point where I have to speak with her about it privately. Raina's biggest complaint is that Alice straightens her room, takes her toothpaste out of the bathroom container and leaves it on the counter "where it gets spit on it from other people," according to Raina, "and, and—"

We finally got Mom to bed after services, and Mom had perhaps her best night's sleep since she's been here. She was asleep by ten. At 3:45 a.m. I noticed the bathroom light on. About five minutes later, the light was shut off, and Mom returned directly to her room and went back to sleep. What's particularly impressive about this is that it is the first time Mom has been able to take the series of steps necessary to get back to her room without turning on and off all lights and entering the wrong rooms. When Mom leaves the bathroom, she has to turn off the bathroom light, which is one of four horizontal switches in a row, but not turn off the night-light, which is another of the four switches. Usually she turns both lights out—or neither. Then she has to turn left (usually she turns right) and walk past Raina's room into her own room. At the entrance to her room, she has to turn off the overhead light for her room, and when she gets into bed, she needs to turn off the lamp on her bedside table. She did all of these and was still sleeping at seven thirty the next morning when I came down to my home office.

Tuesday, October 10

Mom was more alert than usual in the morning. I had thought of inviting her to sit in on my class at some time in the next few weeks and was getting ready to leave when Mom asked where I was going. I said I was leaving to teach my college class in an hour. She asked if she could come, and I said sure. Meanwhile, Ginny came for her first day to begin the transition from Alice to her as the daytime companion. Together they kept Mom company while I handled some errands, and then I returned to pick up Mom and go to class. She remembered where we were going. On the twelve-minute ride, she kept repeating the same questions about the class, but she never forgot that we were going to class.

"How many students do you have?"

"Oh, that many? How do you handle it?"

"How old are they?"

"Oh, one is forty-four years old—how come?"

As with any discussion I have with her, she seemed able to hang onto the main thread but continued to lose almost all information she requested relative to it. So much about this disease is perplexing. I wish I could discern a pattern regarding what Mom does and does not remember. For instance, despite all that she forgets she obviously retains the knowledge that few college students are forty-four years old. Why is this?

During the ninety minutes in class, she sat patiently—as she had in temple—reviewed the written materials, and watched the students interact. During one warm-up activity where students responded to a question about the qualities of an outstanding teacher, she responded in turn. When the students began a group activity, one of the students asked if she'd like to join their group or observe, and she said, "I think I'll just observe, but thank you for asking."

When we got home, we had lunch with Alice and Ginny. Ginny was terrific. She played games with Mom all afternoon:

spelling games, word games, etc. She obviously has a wealth of experience with Alzheimer's patients. Ginny has raised six children of her own, is about fifty, and bubbles with enthusiasm. She will be here every day, Monday through Friday, except for a few Fridays. I'd like to find someone who can be available for occasional evenings or weekends, but hiring Ginny solves our most immediate concern. Ginny wants to net seven dollars an hour. I told her that I would speak with our accountant to determine the best way to accomplish this. I may offer her eight or nine dollars an hour in order for her to get what she needs and for us to able to do it legally and ethically.

I spoke with Laurie Lockwood of Towers Administration, the company providing the long-term care insurance for which my folks had paid monthly premiums since Ed was sixty-five and Mom was fifty-three. There is a $10,000 limit on home health care, each time. We cannot use the policy to pay Ginny because Ginny didn't come from a licensed home care agency. However, if we ever switch to someone from an agency, we can pick up on this policy toward the maximum, or we can go through an agency for weekend and evening supplemental care and take it from the policy. Ginny will charge us between seven and nine dollars an hour; we are still working it out. I'm sure an agency will be much more. The supplementation may work well since it appears that weekends and evenings (when needed) will be our most difficult challenge. Also I learned that if the time comes when Mom has to enter a nursing home, we pay the first thirty days, then we pay 20 percent, and the insurance covers 80 percent up to $150,000.

Sue spoke with Larry. He and Dee have been great. They are still in Florida doing what they can to empty the apartment and settle affairs. We've been in touch with them almost daily (mostly Sue), and they are organizing things for us and will leave relevant information on the table for Gary and me. Larry told Sue that last night they went out to dinner with Millie and Mel, and that Aunt Millie spent the entire first half of the meal complaining of how often Mom called her while Ed was in the hospital. "Two days would be optimistic!" I e-mailed to Gary.

Sue and Larry questioned whether it was wise for me to bring Mom down to Florida just when she was starting to get acclimated to her new home and beginning to rely on Susan, Marli, and Raina along with me. Originally we had thought it might be unfair to Susan to leave her alone with Mom so soon after we had arrived from Florida, but now we aren't sure that would be a problem. I called Gary and told him that if he was comfortable with it, we think it might be better for Mom to stay here. Each day gets a little easier, and she is accepting the situation more comfortably. The fear is that we would be disturbing her routine and disorienting her just when she is starting to become used to our house and to Potsdam. He agreed that maybe I should come down without Mom.

Wednesday, October 11

Today was our best day as far as ease of care. The kids and Sue left for school at seven, and Mom was still sleeping. Ginny arrived at seven thirty and started Mom on an exercise routine when she awoke. Mom and I had some good conversations, and then I was gone from ten o'clock until six this evening. Ginny and Alice took Mom to the Eisenhower locks in Massena. No ships came through, so Ginny might try it again with Mom in the next week or two. They also went walking through the mall before the stores opened. Tonight when I came home, Alice and Mom were playing a dice and word game at the kitchen table. Ginny has been a good influence on Alice. Since Ginny has experience with Alzheimer's patients, she is more proactive with Mom than Alice; she exercises with her and engages her in games and activities. Now Alice is taking the initiative to encourage Mom to play games with her. Tomorrow Mom and I will go to the social security office.

In a phone conversation, Gary suggested Tylenol PM as an alternative to her arthritis pills, and I am glad that he did, or I wouldn't have thought to ask the doctor. In fact, when I called Dr. Kay, he actually took her off her arthritis medicine and gave us another prescription, which he said she shouldn't take right away. "When aches and pains occur," he said, "she should first try Tylenol PM up to four times (eight tablets) a day. If the pains persist, then she should try this new prescription." For at least a few nights, she hasn't needed the Tylenol PM, only the sleeping pills, but I am still glad that Gary suggested it.

Tonight we went out for dinner at a local restaurant—Mom, Raina, Sue, Alice, and me. Mom was delightful company, and we all had a good time. At times she was quite lucid, even recalling details of previous visits to Potsdam. After dinner we went home, and she was quite pleasant but also disoriented. She thought that I was her husband and kept asking why I was sleeping in a different room. When I said I was her son, she wanted to know how many children she had. She indicated that she couldn't find her mother's phone number. When I told her that Grandma had passed away, she was surprised and wanted to know when. When I said it was about twenty-seven years ago, she said, "That long?" We then went through the history of her marriages, starting in 1938. It was a nice conversation, and she was like a good student, thoroughly enjoying the review, punctuating it by telling me, "It's amazing how you remember all those details."

Bedtime and into the early morning hours of the next day were a challenge. Mom awoke around midnight, went into the bathroom, and remained there for over half an hour. Then I heard banging, and I finally got up, walked down the hallway to just outside the bathroom door, and said, "Mom, are you all right?" She shouted through the closed door that the drawer was stuck. I went in and saw her trying futilely to close one of the cabinet drawers. She had been going through drawers, pulling out the kids' jewelry and cosmetics, and looking for who knows what.

I helped her close the drawer and talked her into returning to bed, which she did, and then I returned to the bathroom to put the pilloried jewelry boxes and the girls' drawers back the way they had been before Mom's invasion. Nights like this are to become more frequent, and at times Susan and I feel like we are in a perpetual state of exhaustion.

However, there was a humorous side to this episode. Within five minutes of returning to her bed, and just as I had finished tidying up the bathroom and had started to head back toward my room, Mom was back in the bathroom looking for something else. I guided her to her room again. We repeated this routine twice more before she was once again back in her room, and finally I said, "Mom, it's one in the morning; you have to go to sleep." I put her in bed and turned off her light and returned to my room. Three minutes later her light went on again; this time she was headed past the bathroom, through the gate we had put up to deny her access to the hallway beyond the bathroom door, and she opened Marli's door. I intercepted her before she could enter Marli's room, pointed her toward her room, and repeated, "Mom, it's after one o'clock." She immediately smiled and said, "It's twelve thirty," and she was right. Then she added, "Although that's bad enough."

Hopefully Dr. Kay has received the files from her doctor in Florida, Dr. Levine. I'll call him soon for advice on the sleeping problem. He had told us that the sleeping tablet was temporary, and I need to find out how temporary and what else we can do about the late-night adventures. This seems to be the one difficult hurdle that we need to overcome in order to make Mom's stay manageable.

I am thinking about my meeting with Gary in Florida this coming weekend. Assuming that Mom doesn't go with me, when and how should she travel? Is it desirable, or necessary, to have her return to Florida? Should we take her to visit Gary in North Carolina at some time rather than to Florida? I still have Mom's tickets for Saturday, so if either Gary or Sue has a change of mind, I can take her. Otherwise, I'll extend the time for using the tickets.

Alice, of course, will be returning to her home in Fort Lauderdale this weekend, and, since Mom will probably not be travelling with us, I'm also taking Marli with me to Florida because I think I made a mistake not taking her the last time. She needs to share in the grieving process and the environment. Hopefully we can make a quick visit to the grave site. Beyond that, I think there will be lasting value for her just to be part of the process of making arrangements, visiting Rae, having dinner with Millie and Mel, and joining in some positive and sometimes entertaining experiences with just Gary and me. It's just a gut feeling I have from knowing Marli and from observing what Raina experienced when she was in Florida for Ed's funeral.

Susan reminisces about her mother-in-law:
She was always busy, but it was obvious that when we visited, they put their lives on hold so she could spend all her time with us. They had a very busy and active social life, and she made that happen.

Gail reminisces about her aunt:
The times I remember most are the dinners in Florida with my family at her home, where she seemed most relaxed, and we all enjoyed being together.

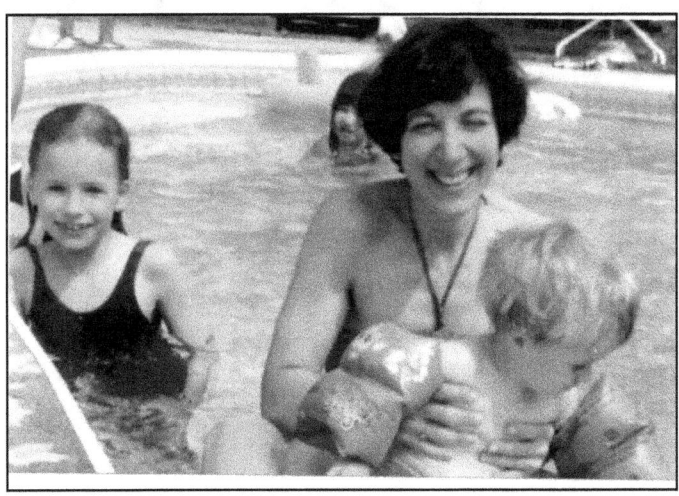

Mom's niece, Gail, holding her son Adam with daughter Rachel next to her in 1988 during visit to Potsdam for Darren's Bar Mitzvah.

Appreciating Mom Through the Lens of Alzheimer's

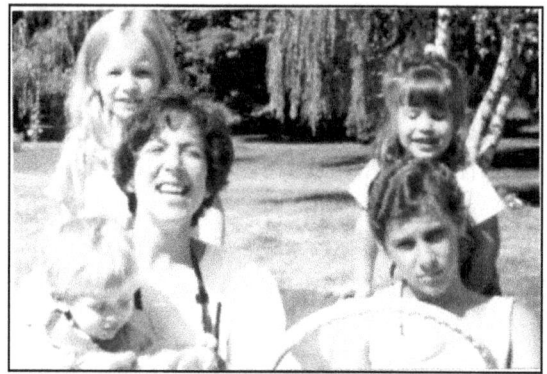

Gail with son Adam on her lap, daughter Rachel behind her alongside of Marli and Darren, 1988.

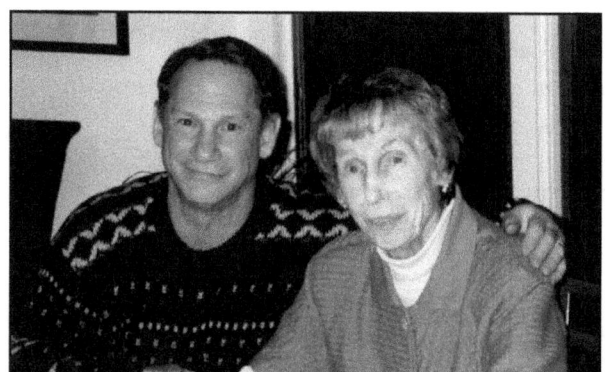

Mom with Don in the fall of 2000 when she began her last eight months living in Potsdam.

Chapter 7

Mom as Elwood P. Dowd

Thursday, October 12

I called Tower Administration in Chicago to find out what Mom is entitled to through her long-term care insurance. I spoke with the boss. He asked me to call back Monday when the lady who can answer our questions will return. He was quite proud of the fact that he had given his employee today and Friday off to attend the White Sox playoff game in Seattle.

I e-mailed Gary that I would fax the lease agreement this afternoon, and that he should ask Laurie to pay particular attention to the last page (the addendum). This is the one that commits Mom and Ed to two years at The Classic.

Today with Mom was wonderful and interesting and presented us with some new problems. She awoke in a very good mood, and after breakfast I took her to the social security office in Ogdensburg, where she made a new friend. Within five minutes Mom learned that the social security representative was born in Heuvelton, ten miles away, is a junior at the local state college while working part time for the social security office, and is currently a science major but is thinking of transferring to a nearby teachers' college. For the first time, she is considering becoming a teacher like her mother, who teaches first grade in the Heuvelton school system, and her father, who is a high school principal.

Mom's new friend had good news for us. As soon as they can process the paper work, Mom's monthly amount will jump from just over five hundred dollars to just under one thousand dollars, retroactive to September. The first payment will include an extra $250 one-time death benefit. If my figuring is correct, Mom should be in pretty decent financial shape for whatever needs there are down the road—at least for the next few years.

It was hell getting Mom to bed tonight. Alice gave her the sleeping pill at eight o'clock, but from eleven to midnight, Mom was out of bed six times, sometimes reentering the bathroom, sometimes wandering into our room, and once wandering into Marli's room. She was always pleasant, often had challenging questions, and was fairly easily redirected back to her own room. At midnight I found her in the bathroom, searching for Tylenol. She said she needed it to go to sleep. After taking two Tylenol PM pills, she returned to her room and slept until eight the next morning.

Sue feels we err if we don't put Mom into bed within ninety minutes of her taking the sleeping pill, as we had done some previous nights. There may be an optimum time to start the bedtime process after the pill has had enough time to take effect—but not too much time. Or maybe some nights we're just luckier than others. We'll find out.

I find that the key to addressing Mom's needs is to take her seriously but to remember that even when she seems lucid and asks reasonable questions like, "Shouldn't I be returning to Florida?" she does not have the same context for what she says or asks as we do. There is a danger of taking her too literally and reacting too seriously. She does not necessarily grasp the meaning of what she says. I don't pretend to understand what she is and is not aware of. For instance, when she asks if she should be returning to Florida, does she grasp the meaning of what she is asking at the time she asks it but then quickly lose the thought and then forget your response? Or is she saying something that is stuck in her memory without ever understanding its meaning, even at the time it is being said? A horse strikes the ground five times if it has been cued to do so when hearing the question, "How old are you?" Does Mom pick up a cue from something someone says that causes her to ask about returning to Florida, without understanding the significance of her question any more than a horse realizes what it means when its foot scratches the surface of the ground five times when asked its age? Or does Mom have a fleeting moment of understanding at the time she poses a question or listens to a response before forgetting it?

Sue and I continued to discuss whether I should take Mom with me to Florida this weekend or let her stay here, but I still have two concerns about leaving her in Potsdam while I fly with Alice to Florida. First, even though we agreed that I should leave Mom in Potsdam, I don't want to deprive Gary of time with Mom. In this regard, I tell Gary that Sue and I will accept whatever he tells us is his honest reaction, but I want him to be candid. Secondly, I continue to worry about placing an undue burden on Sue. I was the only one who could put Mom to bed or calm her anxiety during her first couple of days here. But this is of less concern to me now. She seems to be settling into her new environment, and the furniture and other items around her are becoming familiar; she is becoming accustomed to a schedule that was initially new and disorienting but is rapidly becoming her routine. Clearly she suffered from the newness of everything when she first arrived. As the experts write in books about Alzheimer's sufferers, Mom feels more comfortable when surrounded by familiar items and when ensconced in a routine that is repetitive.

I am also concerned about being away from Mom so soon after we have brought her from Florida because she seems to base her orientation to her surroundings around Gary and me, in a unique way. Part of it is that her memory of other individuals is dependent on who they are in relation to us. "Laurie is Gary's wife; Sue is Don's wife; and the great-grandchild belongs to Brian, who is Gary's son." But part of it is an instinct she seems to have that she can trust us, and if she can't figure something out for herself, security lies in whatever we direct her to do.

So on the one hand, I hate to take Mom away from Potsdam at the very time she is beginning to get into a comfortable, repetitive routine and getting to know her room, its furniture, and its relation to other rooms in the house. However, I am also aware that if she travels with me, she will have a comfort level being with me and then having both Gary and me physically present. I am starting to see, however, that Sue and the kids—particularly Sue—are becoming the same security figures for Mom that Gary and I are. Sue and I are optimistic that it is rapidly reaching the point where it will be almost as easy for Sue to get Mom back to bed or to listen to advice as it has been for Gary and me.

Friday, October 13

Raina is ten years old today, and we celebrated by taking her to dinner at McCarthy's, her favorite restaurant and a preferred choice of local college students for more than fifty years. Raina ordered pasta "with nothing on it—not even that green stuff, just pure white—and with marinara sauce on the side." Mom didn't appear to understand what it means to have a birthday, but she enjoyed the excitement in the air and recognized that this was an event focused on Raina. She had fun playing with the balloon given to Raina by the hostess as we entered.

Gary and I talked to make a final decision on who is going with me to Florida tomorrow. He told me that he is glad that Ginny is into more games and leisure activities as that is a direction he has wanted us to pursue. He thinks it is a good idea to use insurance to cover the more expensive accredited people from an agency for evenings, weekends, and holidays while using Ginny on weekdays and paying her out of pocket. This will preserve a significant amount of insurance for a future time when we may need it. He agreed with my list of agenda items for our brief time in Florida, and he said that he will need to go to the post office as Mom's mail is not being forwarded. He is also having trouble getting his signature accepted on Mom's checks, even though he has a paper giving him power of attorney, so he might have to visit First Union Bank in Florida also. We agree that Marli will go with me to Florida, and Mom will remain in Potsdam with Sue and Raina.

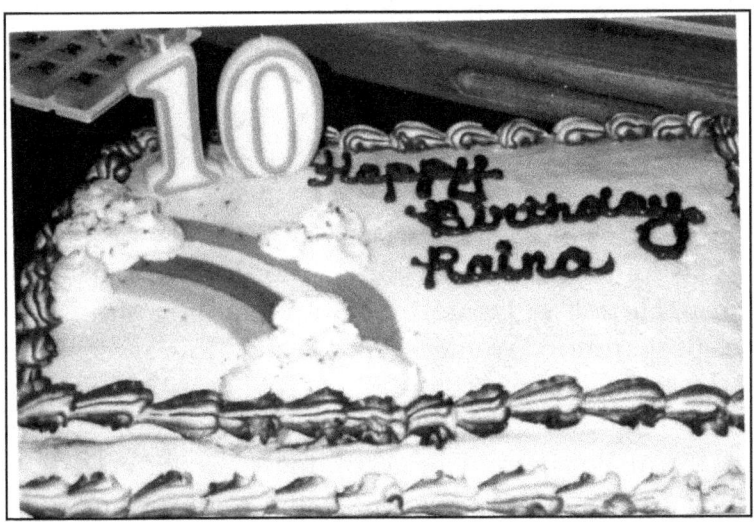

Mom was living in Potsdam in 2000 and was able to celebrate granddaughter Raina's tenth birthday with the family.

Saturday, October 14

Marli, Alice, and I arrived at the West Palm Beach airport in the early evening. Marli and I spent Sunday and part of Monday with Gary, accomplishing most of the items on our list, including going through the apartment and determining what to keep and what to discard. Larry and Dee had already taken what they wanted and had coordinated with us by telephone.

Monday, October 16

Marli and I barely made it on time to the airport for the flight back from Florida, but after that everything went like clockwork. We finally relaxed when we arrived in Syracuse and saw that our luggage had made it also. We were home by eight fifteen. It's Columbus Day weekend, so there was no school today, and that was important to Marli because she does extremely well in school and takes her studies seriously.

Tuesday, October 17

I called Sandra (Mom's Florida broker), and we spoke about Internet access to Mom's account. Gary and I had forgotten to agree on a log-in name, password, and security question, so I told Sandra to use the following:

Log-in: Brian
Password: Marli
Question: Greatest ballplayer
Answer: Willie Mays

I also met with my accountant to discuss transferring records from Florida and to get advice on handling Mom's account and tax preparation. We agreed to allow Mom's accountant in West Palm Beach to finish handling tax-related work through the end of 2000 before transferring records and authorization to my accountant in Potsdam. The accountant also offered a suggestion to protect us in the event that Mom requires nursing home residency for more than three years, which is the amount of time our insurance policy would cover. According to our accountant, if Mom were to be in a nursing home beyond that length of time, once her insurance runs out, they can come after her estate for any monies due. This is not a high probability, but I hear of so many people with stories of Alzheimer's patients who continue their decline for as long as ten years or more. Sue's aunt Hazel is in a hospital bed in a nursing home, where she has been for quite some time. She is unable to communicate, is barely able to move, and is being fed intravenously. The bills can mount quickly, and the accountant is trying to help us anticipate any eventuality.

When I e-mailed this information from the broker and the accountant to Gary, he replied—having been the Giant fan in the family since he was ten—"I appreciate your putting Willie Mays in as part of the code for my sake. A big thanks to you and Marli for all of your help and good cheer in making it a most pleasant and productive weekend."

I called Dr. Kay, and he still hasn't received Mom's medical records. I'll have to call and remind Dr. Levine to send them. Dr. Kay prescribed another round of the sleeping pills. He said not to continue them too long because they can lose effectiveness, and then she will require higher doses. The Tylenol PM can be okay, but he said that it contains Benadryl, which can also act as a stimulant.

Sue is going to try cutting Mom's dose back to half a pill a night. There's no specific timetable the doctor could give us. He just suggested that "gradually" it will require higher dosages to accomplish the same effect if we give her the sleeping pill on a regular basis. Also, Mom complains frequently about an upset stomach. We have our next appointment in early November, and Dr. Kay said that he would give her a thorough examination then to make sure there are no other serious problems causing her erratic sleeping habits. He said that they could easily be caused by stress related to her condition or Ed's passing, but that he wanted to make sure it's not a tumor or some such thing.

Thursday, October 19

Blanche Jimenez is a colleague from Queens, New York, who has been a staff developer, teacher, principal, and fellow board member of The Institute for Learning Centered Education, an organization I founded in 1994. She learned of Mom's condition from a mutual friend and sent us this e-mail:

> My mother had Alzheimer's too! It's not easy—just think of the times before your mom had it. Every once in a while I remember how my mother, although she stopped talking, would wink her eye, just like the old days when she could have a cigarette dangling out of her mouth, wash dishes, and talk to me about Isaac Asimov's latest science fiction novel all at the same time. My heart goes out to you, Susan, and the kids.

Appreciating Mom Through the Lens of Alzheimer's

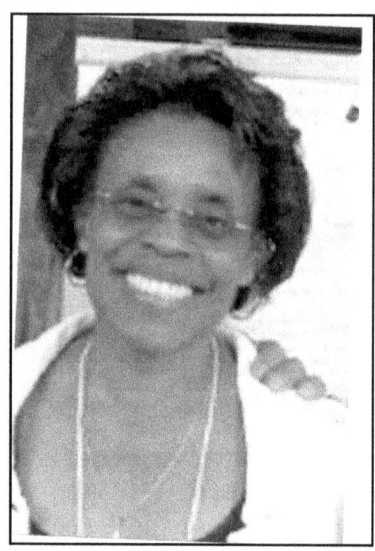

Blanche Jimenez, a colleague and friend whose mother had passed away with Alzheimer's. "It's not easy," she wrote.

Saturday, October 21

Late in the morning, we decided to take Mom to the mall (a forty-minute drive) for shopping. We thought that she would enjoy walking through the stores as well as the chance to people watch in the corridors. So the five of us went to the mall to shop for clothes and boots for Mom. We arrived at noon, and Raina and Mom grabbed a table and chatted for thirty minutes as I waited in lines at the food court, and Marli and Sue shopped. Mom had a turkey sub with lettuce and tomato. When I asked her if she wanted anything else on it, she asked me if I thought catsup would be good. I suggested mayo instead, and she took my advice.

Recently Sue said that one reason she was sure Raina would love having Grandma around was because Grandma, in her current condition, would become the younger sister Raina didn't have. Wow, was that prophetic—as it began on the plane ride from Florida to Syracuse, that's exactly what has happened. I've also decided that Mom is Elwood P. Dowd reincarnated: always pleasant, friendly with anyone who will respond to a smiling hello, and always cheerful—just like the character in the play whose imaginary friend, Harvey, was a six-foot-one-inch white rabbit. As the five of us wandered through the Bon Ton, Mom stopped at every dancing stuffed animal, sang along with it, and commented with a giggle, "Isn't that cute? Did you see that Santa Claus dancing to 'Holly Jolly Christmas?'"

We passed a check-out counter, and the lady smiled at Mom, so Mom gave her a big "Hello, how are you?" In a moment, they were chatting like old friends. I half expected Mom, as Elwood, to say, "Here, let me give you my card!" or "Why don't you come to our house for dinner?" or "May I introduce you to my friend, Harvey?" The lady said, "It's a bit early for winter, but you may even have to drive home in oh." At least it sounded like "oh." Mom laughed heartily, and as we walked away, she asked me, "What did she say?" This was not a result of her dementia. The lady didn't pronounce the last word clearly, and I had to struggle to figure out that she meant "snow." But Mom wanted to reinforce her, so she laughed when she knew a laugh was expected. When I clarified for Mom, she said, "Oh, I thought she said 'You may even have to drive home in oh.' I didn't hear her say snow."

Throughout our walk among the stores, Mom stopped at everything a four-year-old would find appealing. It was refreshing to see her appreciation of things simple and pretty. In one conversation yesterday, she recalled exactly what Darren is doing, that he is in real estate. Usually she asks about how he's doing in college and completely forgets everything else about him. On the other hand, yesterday she also kept looking for our third daughter. This is characteristic: surprisingly accurate pieces of reality mixed with confusion about other aspects.

We shopped in several stores and got Mom some boots and warm clothes. Periodically she suggested that we not spend any money on her since "I won't be here long." Sometimes I said, "Well, even if it's only one day of snow, you need the boots." Other times I reminded her that, "Our home is your home now, and you'll be with us all winter." She accepted this, for the moment.

Sometimes I reminded her, "Ed passed away, and you need to be with family now." Then she would say either "He did? When?" or "That's right, I forgot."

We arrived home around four o'clock; she napped for twenty minutes; we had dinner, and then Mom and Raina watched *Cat Ballou*, a favorite of Raina's. Sue and I drove Marli to her high school dance then returned and watched a different movie in another room.

Susan reminisces about her mother-in-law:
The quality I admired most in her was her love of life. It was always easy for her to make friends because she was so interested in people, always asking questions, and truly interested in what she was hearing.

Gail reminisces about her aunt:
The quality I remember the most was her ability to listen and to be interested and to hear.

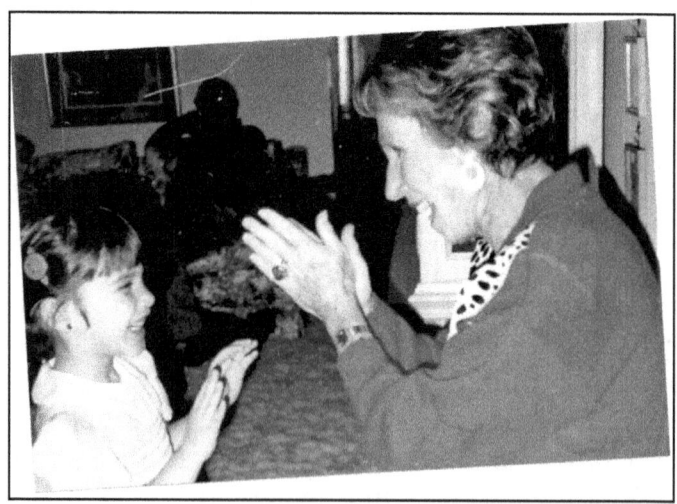

Marli and Mom play pat-a-cake.

Chapter 8

The Family Tree Sparks Memories

Sunday, October 22

I napped in the afternoon, which is highly unusual for me because I have rarely in my life, even as a child, been tired enough to fall asleep at any time other than bedtime. Sue took Mom into town and to several stores for a few hours, and she was fine. We all had a nice dinner together. After dinner, Raina worked with her grandmother, drawing a chart of our family tree. She did this after Mom kept asking who her children were. Sometimes she said that she has three children, and as is typical, the disorientation seemed to increase with the lateness of the hour. When Mom insisted for the third time that she has three children, Raina informed her, "You have two children, Grandma—Gary and Don." Raina then led Mom in a discussion of who Darren, Brian, Sally, Todd, and Katie are in relation to her.

"Where does Brian live?" Mom asked.

"Charlotte, North Carolina," Raina responded.

"And is he married?"

"Yes, he and Sally just had your first great-grandchild."

"Oh, that's right. And where does Todd live?"

"Michigan."

"And is Todd married?"

"Todd and Katie are engaged and will be getting married in Minnesota next May."

Finally Raina put together the written tree, and Mom really liked this.

"When did Ed die?" she asked.
"A month ago," Raina answered.
"What was the date?"
"September 28."
Mom wrote, "Died September 28" next to Ed's name on the tree.
"How old was Harold when he died?" she asked.
"Fifty-two," Raina answered.
Mom wrote, "Died at 52" next to Harold on the tree.
At eight o'clock we went upstairs and watched a tape of Darren's Bar Mitzvah. Mom enjoyed seeing Rae and Lenny, Gary and Laurie, and others she could identify. At 8:45 p.m. we turned off the VCR and sent Raina to bed. Mom said, "Tomorrow, let's talk about when I'm going home."
"Mom, you are home."
"But maybe I should go home to Long Island."
"Mom, you haven't lived on Long Island for thirty years."
"But don't my mother and sister need me?"
"Mom, they haven't lived on Long Island for thirty years. Grandma passed away, and Aunt Millie is living in Florida with Mel."
At bedtime we gave her half of the sleeping pill that Dr. Kay had prescribed. Her bedtime routine took two hours, and Sue suggested once again that we start it no later than eight thirty in the future. By eleven o'clock Mom was in bed. She went right to sleep and slept until seven thirty the next morning. I don't know if the sleeping pill—as opposed to the Tylenol PM—helps her get a better night's sleep, or if she's just destined to have a bad night every three or four nights. Or, maybe it will get better as she gets more oriented to this house. Other than at bedtime, there are definitely signs of improvement as Mom grows familiar with the house and a daily routine. She finds things more easily, goes straight to her own room more frequently, and seems more comfortable.

Monday, October 23

Tonight was tough. Mom, Raina, and I watched a tape of Marli's Bat Mitzvah. Then at eight thirty we gave Mom the half pill, as we had done the night before when it had worked so well. But tonight she went through the same routine at least five times between eleven o'clock and three. She opened the door to her room, walked the fifteen feet to the bathroom, and closed the bathroom door. Periodically, either Sue or I walked down the hallway and asked, "Are you okay, Mom?" Eventually she opened the door, but when she emerged, sometimes she turned left and went straight into her room; other times she turned right and headed toward our room, and we had to redirect her. Each time, within a few minutes of entering her room, she reemerged and headed back into the bathroom. Finally at three o'clock, she went into her room; Sue got her into bed, and she fell asleep.

Half an hour later, while Sue and I were asleep, she woke up again, walked out of her room, entered the bathroom, and started emptying the drawers. When I finally awoke and noticed her in the bathroom, I got out of bed and gently took her hand. As I was leading her back to her room, she said, "Ed must be missing me. When are you taking me home, Don?"

"You are home, Mom. This is your home now."

"It is?" she responded.

"Yes, Ed passed away a month ago."

"Oh, that's right. This is my home now?"

"Yes."

"Who else lives here?"

"Raina, Marli, and Sue."

"Oh, how long have you lived here?"

"More than four years in this particular house."

"That long—I didn't know that."

I tucked her into her bed, said good night, and returned to my room. However, by this time I couldn't sleep, so I went down to the computer and prepared for my Tuesday morning class. I also reflected on her comment that Ed must be missing her. What does this mean? Is she thinking that he is at home in Florida waiting for her? Does she feel any emotion about not being with him?

Wednesday, October 25

Mom slept better last night, and she is eating much better lately. Complaints of headaches and stomachaches are fewer. Alice called to see how Mom is doing, but Mom was out. When they returned from a quick trip into town, Sue helped Mom call, and she and Alice talked for a while.

Thursday, October 26

I received the letter from Dr. Kay that Laurie had requested to help us get out of the two-year lease agreement with The Classic. It's very brief—possibly too brief:

"Rhoda Meister is an 83-year-old woman who has recently moved to Potsdam to the residence of her son following the death of her husband. Due to deterioration in her health, she is not able to live independently and can no longer be expected to live in the apartment where they had been residing."

I immediately put it in the mail for Laurie, with a note indicating that if it is not sufficient, she should let me know, and I will ask him to rewrite it and add more detail. I wouldn't ask him to write anything that isn't factual, but there could be things that need to be in the letter that are true, which he did not think to include.

Gary and I will probably need to make one more trip to Florida in November or December to help clean out the apartment, make decisions, and tend to other details. On another note, my stockbroker in Potsdam, Joe, is checking with a jewelry expert to advise us on our options for selling some of Mom's jewelry. He said that we should be prepared that we may not be able to get close to the appraised value.

I decided to write to the Fitzgeralds in Jacksonville, Florida. Donald Fitzgerald worked as an attorney in the same Maryland office of the Department of Agriculture that my dad did. He and his wife, Leilani, a nutritionist, and my parents were close friends. Donald and Leilani have since moved to Jacksonville, where Leilani continues to work full time, and he does part-time consulting.

In my e-mail, I told them that "Mom and Dad were always so fond of you, and Mom spoke highly of you as being there more than anyone else after my dad passed away. Mom and Ed enjoyed every visit to you, usually late June, for so many years as they would wend their way up to Potsdam through Jacksonville and Chapel Hill for their summer visits with us." I told them that Mom is in the early to mid-stages of Alzheimer's, and I added, "While it's not true of all Alzheimer's patients, Mom retains her wonderful, pleasant, and optimistic disposition. At times she's quite lucid, and at other times we have to remind her (a dozen times in ten minutes) of who we are and who she knows. But, as our son, Darren, said when he visited her in Florida in September, 'Dad, no matter how confused or frustrated Grandma gets, she's always smiling and cheerful.'"

Gary called and commiserated over the dilemma of taking Mom off the sleeping pills and having to deal with her restlessness at night. He asked if we still have the marks on the doors to help her identify her room and if we are encouraging her to use them when she goes back to her room from the bathroom. He thinks the family tree is a great idea, and he encouraged us to get her to refer to it when she asks questions rather than answering them for her. "If you can encourage her to use all of the visual cues you are setting up," he said, "she might start to do that more automatically."

I responded, "Yes, we have the doors labeled. Your idea about getting her to use the cues rather than giving them ourselves is excellent. It's probably similar to the reason we train teachers to challenge their students to answer their own questions rather than rely on the teacher for all the answers. You have suggested this previously—good advice—and we have been trying to do that."

The problem is not so much that Mom goes to the wrong room anymore, although that was a problem when she first arrived. It is more that when she gets into the bathroom she becomes disoriented, starts searching for things, uses the kids' toothbrushes, empties drawers, and leaves everything from towels to toilet paper strewn around the floor and over the sink. By the time she comes out—sometimes as much as forty-five minutes after she entered the bathroom—she has forgotten whose house she is in or even if she wants to, or should, return to bed. The situation is improving a little because now when she finally does come out of the bathroom, she will often find her room, using some of the cues, but then she is back out in another minute to return to the bathroom. So at least we are making progress. She is going to the right places more often.

Gary and I agreed that we should probably both go down later in November or in December, when we can stay for a few days if necessary. That might work better than trying to squeeze too much into a shorter stay before then, and hopefully we can tie up loose ends and finally close things down. Also, by that time we should be able to see if we can locate someone to buy the furniture; we will have decided what to do with their car; and we will be in a better position to finalize things.

Friday, October 27

Ginny wasn't able to come in today, so I had to wake Mom at seven thirty so she could accompany me to Syracuse, two and a half hours away. Actually, this was about the only day since Mom has been here that anyone has had to wake her. Every other day we would let her sleep until she awoke on her own—usually around eight or eight thirty. At seven thirty I knocked on her door, then yelled in a few times. Just like with a teenager, she asked, "Can I sleep a little longer?" I woke her again at 7:45, and we left the house at 8:55—ten minutes later than planned—and stopped at McDonald's for breakfast fifteen minutes into our trip.

She really enjoyed McDonald's—got her standard Egg McMuffin without the meat, decaf coffee (she has to be reminded that she can't have caffeine), and five pills that I had brought with us. Mom was in a super mood. She sat in the car and kept finding the one speck of blue in the sky and repeatedly observed, "I think it's trying to clear up."

Traveling for the next two hours was fine. She catnapped only once or twice, sat quietly for stretches, seemed to enjoy the music, even sang along to a Peggy Lee song, and frequently commented about how it was trying to clear up. Often she asked where we were going. "How much longer will it be?" Each time we heard the weather forecast, she acted astonished that it was going to turn much colder the next day. In short, we had a delightful trip.

My meeting was at Syracuse University with two colleagues. Mom had a warm smile for them as they were introduced, sat quietly as we talked, ordered bring-in lunch with us, and ate a whole turkey sandwich on pita. To my colleagues Mom probably appeared to be a perfectly normal, healthy woman. In fact, when I exited for a pit stop and returned five minutes later, the three of them were engaged in animated conversation. Mom was asking questions and showing an interest in their responses, none of which was surprising. We got home at six o'clock (she barely slept on the return trip), had a quick dinner, went to temple, came home, and after the usual seventy-five minute routine, Mom went to bed. She stayed asleep until two thirty, got up to go to the bathroom, returned to her room a while later, and slept until nine.

Saturday, October 28

This morning, as usual, Mom was cheerful. She joined the four of us for breakfast and then headed off at noon for the mall with Susan. They went to buy Mom a warm nightgown, do grocery shopping, and run a few errands, probably returning around five o'clock. This was my chance to get some work done. I usually rely on having Sunday mornings to do work while everyone else is at temple. Susan, as principal of the Sunday school, takes Mom to temple when her vice principal is there because the vice principal enjoys having Mom sit in on her classes and can handle it. Unfortunately, the vice principal has been out the last two weeks, so in anticipation of spending tomorrow morning with Mom, I was getting my work done this afternoon.

The times I have alone with Mom are enjoyable. Tomorrow while Susan and Raina are in temple, we'll probably clean the fish tanks together and maybe go to McDonald's for breakfast. In short, we're doing fine. Evenings are still the major hurdle, although they are gradually getting better. There doesn't seem to be any pattern we can spot as to when Mom sleeps well and when she's up, on and off, for three or four hours. It doesn't seem to correlate to how active or inactive she's been during the day nor to whether she has the sleeping pill, or half a pill, or the Tylenol PM. There doesn't seem to be a direct correlation to whether she has napped during the day or had a good night's sleep the previous night.

As Gary had observed in Florida in September, Mom is clearly more alert in the mornings. She seems as likely to mistake people or be in a different period of her life in the morning as later, but the major difference I notice is that her mood is brighter, her outlook cheerier, the earlier in the day it is. Her disorientation (and concern) grows with the passing of the day. She is much more likely to ask when she is going home in the afternoon—particularly after dinner—and to stay on that topic the later it is in the day. Earlier in the day, her focus is more on who and what is happening around her. After dinner, it is more on where is she, how will she get her belongings up here (the ones to which she refers are already here), and whether she should call Millie, Rae, or whomever else she fixates on for the moment. We continue to look for patterns—a few are emerging, but not many, and none that we can see in terms of forecasting how well she will sleep or what we can do about it.

Leilani Fitzgerald called this morning. She started out by describing her heart attack, which occurred last Sunday, and she said she took two aspirins, was rushed to the hospital, took and passed a stress test on Wednesday, and was home by Thursday, feeling fine. I told her it sounded like listening to someone describe a routine cold.

They hadn't heard of Ed's passing—or Lenny's, for that matter—until receiving my e-mail. I filled her in, and then she spoke with Mom for about ten minutes. Mom unintentionally laid some guilt trips on her as she kept repeating, "It's been so long since I've heard from you."

Sunday, October 29

This afternoon, Mom received this e-mail from Leilani:

"Hello Rhoda, it was good talking with you on the phone today. Donald and I are so thankful that Don got in touch with us through e-mail. We would never want to lose touch with you or your family. You have been an integral part of our lives for over thirty-five years, and that fact is important to us.

"Don caught us up on what is happening to you. We are so sorry to learn of Ed's passing. We know how hard this time must be for you. We are glad that you are with Don and his family. I can close my eyes and still see Ed sitting at the end of our dining room table, the very first time we met him. We were so happy for you that you had him in your life. We never forgot Harold, and we still talk about him, especially his capacity to tell a story about an incident or something. He would start turning circles with his index fingers. The deeper he got into his story, the tighter the circles would become, until the index fingers would circle each other, barely touching. You have been truly blessed to have such wonderful men to share your life with, your husbands and your sons, and now all your grandchildren.

"Let's see if I can catch you up on some of the news from our end. I caused some excitement last weekend by having a heart attack. I told Don about it on the phone, so he can catch you up on the details. The thought has crossed my mind that maybe Ed was communicating subliminally with me, telling me what to do, because the doctors and nurses commented many times that I did all the little things correctly for the successful outcome. Of course there are really good drugs that are available now, but if you do not do things right, you are not a candidate for these drugs. I am fine now. So much for that news. Leilani & Don"

I forwarded the e-mail to Gary, who responded, "How nice and sweet. Brought tears to my eyes. Thanks so much for sending it along. I don't remember the part about Dad circling with his fingers at all—probably never noticed it myself. Do you remember that?"

I had some tears, too, when I read Leilani's e-mail, but I don't recall the circling fingers either. I suggested to Gary that "Dad may have acted differently in his own social circles (pun intended) than when he would share stories and information with us."

Monday, October 30

Mom is finding her room better, but her sleeping habits continue to be erratic. She can stay in the bathroom, and does, for thirty to forty-five minutes at a time. She seems to sleep well every other or every third night. One night she will get into bed at ten thirty, be back in the bathroom at midnight, and be there on and off until three. However, from the time she gets into bed until 3:00 a.m., she can make round trips to the bathroom six or more times.

From three o'clock on, she seems to sleep well and usually doesn't get up until eight or eight thirty. If she does get up between three and eight, it is to go the bathroom, and she returns right to bed without any interventions from us.

Marli and Raina have adjustments to make that are different from the changes required of Susan and me, due to the effects of living with and caring for Mom. They are the ones sharing their bathroom with her. When Mom disappears into the bathroom for forty-five minutes at a time, they have no access to their toiletries and therefore must go into our room (if our door is open) or downstairs if they need to use the facility. Also it is their combs, brushes, cosmetics, jewelry, toothbrushes, and other possessions that end up almost anywhere upstairs after one of Mom's rummaging explorations.

Raina reminisces about her grandmother:
I always looked forward to being with Grandma because she was always so nice and sweet, making it always nice to be around her.

Susan reminisces about her mother-in-law:
I remember her enjoyment with both of our daughters when we were visiting in Florida and we would go to a show or restaurant where they could dress up. I also remember when Marli was much younger and before Raina was born how much she enjoyed and played with Marli and Adam during the summer of Darren's Bar Mitzvah (1988). They were both in diapers, and she loved sitting with them at the shallow end of the pool while Gail and I enjoyed some quiet time.

The Family Tree Sparks Memories

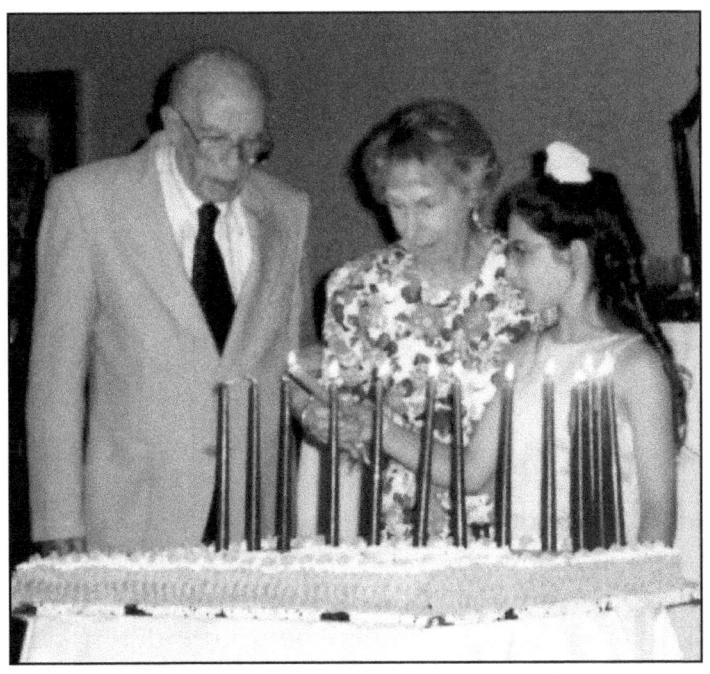

Ed, Mom and Marli participate in a candle lighting ritual during Marli's Bat Mitzvah August 16, 1987.

Chapter 9

Rapid Deterioration: "I Wish I Could Die"

Wednesday, November 1

Ginny said Mom was particularly disoriented today—couldn't handle the usual Scrabble words, wasn't sure what the word "shower" meant. There may be a little deterioration. She seems to have trouble, occasionally, with words that she used to understand easily.

Thursday, November 2

Mom seemed to be having a good day. Ginny played games with her and took her into town to observe as Ginny had her hair done. Then Mom decided that she wanted hers done too, so they both had their hair done by Ginny's hairdresser. Mom usually gets her hair done every other week by another hairdresser, the one Sue goes to.

At three thirty this afternoon, she decided to take a nap but kept coming out of her room every three minutes, and we had the same repetitious dialogue:

"Mom, I thought you were going to nap?"

"I am. I just need to get something from the bathroom. What time is dinner?"

"We'll leave here about five thirty and go over to the university for an informal meal. They have a nice buffet with a wide selection of foods."

"Will you wake me?"

"Yes, I'll wake you forty-five minutes before we have to leave."

"Good."

This cycle repeated itself for almost an hour. Then Sue arrived home from school, and I went out for a while. When I came back to pick them all up at five thirty, Mom was ready but still hadn't napped. She ate a good meal and seemed to enjoy looking at all the tables filled with students. At seven thirty I took out the *Family Play* movie that Fred had directed and taped the week after Darren's Bar Mitzvah in 1988. Most of the family came to Potsdam for the event and turned it into an extended family vacation. Brian, Todd, and Darren as teenagers and Marli as a toddler are featured, but there are good shots of Ed, Kip, Millie, Susan, Gail, Adam, Mom, and Rachel. Mom really enjoyed it. Over the next few months, we will watch this tape many times, and it becomes Mom's favorite, probably because it includes her and most of us who were closest to her—the other six of us remaining from the family of ten who shared so many happy meals together, our spouses, and those of our children who had been born at that time.

She then took her usual seventy-five minutes to get ready for bed—most of it in the bathroom. Then I walked her to her room. As she sat on the edge of her bed, she became quite serious, spoke in a normal, though depressed, tone, and said sadly, "Don, I just don't feel right any of the time."

"What's wrong, Mom?"

"Nothing feels right. I have nothing to live for; it's not going to get better."

"I know it's not easy, Mom."

"No, it's not."

"Well, we have a doctor's appointment next week. Maybe he can suggest something."

"There's nothing he can do. What can he suggest? I'm alone. It's not going to get better. I just don't feel right. Nothing feels right. It's like this all the time."

"Well, maybe the doctor will have something to suggest."

"There's nothing anyone can do. I wish I could just die."

"Get a good night's sleep, Mom, that's the best thing for you right now."

"What time do I have to get up?"

"Eight thirty."

"You'll wake me?"

"I'll wake you."

"I'd be better off if I could just die."

"Mom, you're usually the one who's the optimist."

"There's nothing to be optimistic about."

"You need to get some sleep, you haven't slept well the last couple of nights, you didn't nap much today."

"What time do I have to get up?"

"Eight thirty."

"You'll wake me?"

"I'll wake you, good night! I love you."

"I love you too."

Was this a rare time these thoughts entered her consciousness, or does she have thoughts like these often, but only occasionally articulates them?

Friday, November 3

I'm trying to get a complete folder to the accountant and broker of everything related to Mom's finances. I asked Gary to please forward the latest copies of the brokerage account statements and Treasury Bonds' statements from Mom's Florida broker when he gets a chance.

Ginny said that Mom has been much better yesterday and today—a lot less of the disorientation she experienced on Wednesday.

Susan has an ally in Mom for going to temple every Friday; I used to be able to get away with going once every month or two. Now it's, "Your mom really wants to go to temple." And it's true. Mom really lights up at the thought of going to temple; it must represent security, familiarity, a reminder of childhood, or something like that. We have been to temple just about every Friday evening since she's been here.

It continues to be fun to watch Raina and Mom interact. Raina was a big help tonight, guiding Mom through her prolonged bedtime ritual between the bedroom and bathroom and back. Since there is no school tomorrow, we were able to let Raina stay with Mom until the ritual was just about over; whereas, we normally have to cut Raina's role short on school nights. Of course, Raina participated in keeping Mom on task eagerly, since for Raina, the alternative is earlier to bed.

Saturday, November 4

We watched Mom's favorite tape of Fred's *Family Play* from the week of Darren's Bar Mitzvah again the other night. Gail was trying to hit a baseball without too much luck, and every time she swung and missed, Mom exclaimed, "Oh!" She was rooting for Gail to succeed and obviously understood the difference between success and failure with a baseball bat and ball.

Gary wants me to ask Dr. Kay to revise his letter, giving reasons why Mom can't be expected to handle assisted living at The Classic. He said Laurie thinks that the letter must include more details on the exact nature of Mom's disabilities at this stage of her affliction, so I e-mailed Gary that I would request it and will forward it as soon as it arrives.

Overall, this week has gone better. Mom slept very well Tuesday, Wednesday, and Thursday nights—sleeping until about nine thirty the first two and awakening at eight thirty on Friday morning. Of course when I commented to Susan Thursday morning on how well Mom had slept the night before, her response was, "You mean *you* slept very well."

"Why, was Mom was up in the middle of the night?" I asked.

"At least three times that I got up with her," she replied. "Didn't you wake up when she walked into our room?"

Nevertheless, Mom does sleep much later than usual and is more "with it" during the days than at any time recently. Thursday night neither Susan nor I was awakened by Mom nor saw her get up, but Susan indicated that there is some evidence of her rummaging through the bathroom.

Sunday, November 5

Gary spent the last of three days in Nottingham, England, giving presentations for parents and professionals on autism, and he was at the airport getting ready to board a flight home when he e-mailed me. "No sign of Robin Hood or Maid Marian yet, but I am still looking. Hope you all had a good week. Where are you off to for Thanksgiving, or are you staying home?"

As it is only two days before what would turn out to be one of the most controversial presidential elections in the history of our country, I replied, "Maid Marian and Robin Hood are in Florida, trying to take ballots from the rich and give them to Al Gore."

I also told Gary that we will be heading to Sue's sister Alice's home in Briarcliff Manor in a few weeks for Thanksgiving. Mom will have a basement bedroom and bathroom, and Sue and I will also sleep in the basement in a room just outside Mom's. The door to her room opens into ours, and there is a bathroom easily accessible to both rooms. I'm going to try to get Mom out to the Long Island cemetery where Mom's parents and our dad are buried and to the School Street houses, possibly on Friday when the rest of the family heads for the city.

I concluded the e-mail, informing Gary that I have opened a brokerage account for her in Potsdam and asked if he could send a check from the Fidelity account in Florida either to me or directly to the broker in Potsdam for deposit.

Gary e-mailed back: "Sounds like a big job handling Mom, and I certainly appreciate all of your efforts as well as Sue's and the rest of the family's. I know it won't be easy under any circumstances, but improving the sleep situation would certainly help. What about not letting her sleep so late? Might be harder for that day, but do you think she might sleep better in the long run?" He closed his e-mail by saying that he just got called to board his plane.

I responded: "There are rewards that outweigh any difficulties. I really appreciate all that you are handling, that you were able to get down to Florida a couple of times while Ed was in the hospital when it would have been difficult for us to get away, and that you are handling the finances and so many of the details. I think we have a good team effort going." I responded to his suggestion by saying that we haven't seen any correlation between how early or late she rises and how easily she retires the next night.

Monday, November 6

Helen Lobell, a longtime friend of Mom's, called today. She wasn't aware that Ed had passed away and has been trying to reach them through The Classic.

Fred sent an e-mail to Mom. She has never worked on a computer, so I printed the message and read it to her. "Dear Aunt Rhoda, My campaign for the city council is going well. Lots of people tell me I have a good chance. Win or lose, I will be happy. Carole is taking a course on creative writing in the English department and enjoys it very much. She is still trying to get her novel published. We all miss you. Love, Fred."

As more people learn of Mom's condition, additional friends and colleagues are motivated to send us their thoughts. I received the following from the superintendent of a very small school district in Newcomb, New York, for whom I had conducted staff development workshops.

"Dear Don, After my mom could no longer verbalize her thoughts or even assure us she knew us, she smiled and KISSED! The need for social contact was there, and like a baby who would not remember the early months later in life, at the time they know how they feel. At the end, I crawled into bed with Mom to hug her—it had been so long since someone had slept by her and hugged her! Teaching and learning is listening to some of your better human instincts. Regards, Barbara Kearns."

Saturday, November 11

This was my birthday, and Gail sent me a warm greeting and included this note to Mom: "Hi Aunt Rhoda, I am busy doing my university counseling and my private practice. This is a very busy time since lots of students need counseling what with leaving home, taking exams, etc. We are all fine. We are going to Florida to visit my mother and Mel on December 26. We will miss seeing you. I hope that you are nicely settled in now. Much love to you and all the Mesibovs from all of us!"

For my birthday Susan, the girls, Mom, and I traveled to Lake Placid, a ninety-minute ride, for a nice dinner at an excellent Italian restaurant. We then went to a local theatrical production of *The Miracle Worker*. I was curious to see how Mom would handle this since it was the first time in a while she wouldn't begin bedtime preparations at eight thirty. She handled everything beautifully. She enjoyed dinner and sat quietly and attentively through the production. At the end of the second act, she asked if it was over. When it was over, she asked if there would be more and indicated dissatisfaction that we wouldn't find out how it ended, even though we just did. She was talkative on the ride home (arrived at 11:35 p.m.) and then took her usual seventy-five minutes to prepare for bed.

Sunday, November 12

Mom was up by eight o'clock this morning, and so far it is a typical day.

Tuesday, November 14

Gary called and said that he had a brief phone discussion with the agent from The Classic yesterday. It was quite interesting, he said, and there was a surprise wrinkle. The Classic people think Mom can make it in their assisted care unit as long as she is not violent and does not fall. They said they have a number of dementia clients there. He suggested that this gives us another option to consider. He also said that Laurie is reviewing the lease again to see how this fits in and if we still want to get out of it.

Wednesday, November 15

I e-mailed Gary that I knew this was an option; Aunt Millie had pushed this the time I met with her right after Ed's death. I just feel that Mom is better off in the situation where we have her now. I pointed out that the only thing she has left is that she recognizes us, as family. Even though at times she can't even place us, she gets security and comfort from being around us and our constant interaction. I can't believe that she would get the same involvement, security, and mental stimulation in an assisted living home. Once she no longer has recognition of any of us, or if her physical abilities deteriorate to the point where we can't care for her, I could see considering an assisted living or nursing home option. We have one here in Canton, and Gary has mentioned one in Chapel Hill; I have been thinking that either of them will be possibilities when the time comes and we need to.

"But what would Mom have in Florida?" I asked. At first she'd get periodic visits from Aunt Millie and Rae, but these would take up less than 1 percent of the time that she has people around her here in Potsdam. As they find it more and more frustrating to be with her, their visits and those of any friends would diminish. Aunt Millie has already gone from calling almost daily during the first week after we brought Mom here to not calling at all and sometimes not returning a call from Mom for a few days. Rae has called twice; Helen Lobell called once; and no one else has called at all. "Who's going to visit her if she's in Florida?" I asked. I am certain she will go weeks at a time without seeing anyone from outside the assisted living facility except Gary's family and us, when we come down for whatever visits we can make.

Here she is being exercised every morning, spends the day with Ginny, plays games, goes for walks—even on cold days—goes shopping with Sue and on day trips with the family most weekends, and plays Scrabble and other games with Sue and the kids regularly. Raina has made her a huge poster-board chart of the family tree with pictures of Gary, Laurie, Brian, Todd, and the rest of us, and Raina and Marli go over it with her daily.

Little of this would happen in the best of nursing or assisted living homes. I concluded by asking Gary if he has explored with the representative what The Classic feels are the options if Mom does not go into their assisted living facility. I suggested that it is possible that they won't contest releasing Mom from the lease regardless of what they feel are their legal rights, particularly if there are plenty of buyers out there.

Thursday, November 16

Mom's appointment with Dr. Kay is tomorrow. Ginny is going to take her since I have a meeting at the time of her appointment, and I don't want to postpone the appointment.

Friday, November 17

Gary has commented a number of times about my observations of how much Mom enjoys looking at pictures of all of us, seeing the video Fred directed, and talking on the phone with people she feels close to. He said that when everyone in his family gathers at his home over Thanksgiving, he will try to organize some regular telephone calls to Mom. He joked, "It won't be long before Anna is ready to call on a regular basis as well."

I responded that I think this is a good idea; Mom really enjoys the phone calls she gets. Sue urges me to suggest that maybe if each close relative could pick a different night of the week and try to call Mom weekly on that evening, it would give Mom continuity. We could build up her expectations for a particular person each day with photographs and discussion.

Gary also said that Laurie thinks that we should know our legal rights before broaching the question with The Classic about whether we have the right to end the lease, and I agree with him. We will delay pursuit of that until Laurie receives the revised letter from Dr. Kay and until she can render her opinion.

I'm still trying to figure out how Mom's brain is affected by this affliction. For instance, how come she can't remember answers, but she keeps remembering and repeating the same questions? Once she asks a cycle of questions, she repeats the cycle and rarely shifts to a different set of questions. (Example: Where are we going? How far is it? When are we eating? Where are we going? How far is it? When are we eating? Where are we going?) Why is it that almost all of Mom's questions have to do with what comes next? Is this typical of most Alzheimer's sufferers, or do they all have different patterns?

We contacted a caregivers' agency, who will send in someone for a few hours each weekend or to cover us any night as the need arises. Towers Administration will cover the cost, which is fifteen dollars per hour.

Ginny took Mom to her appointment with Dr. Kay today, and I gave her a note to remind him that we need a more detailed letter explaining why Mom would not be able to handle assisted living.

Sunday, November 19

An hour before the children and Sue left for Sunday school, Mom and I got in the car and headed for the mall. As soon as we pulled out of the driveway, Mom noticed how wet the roads were. I told her that the roads were wet because the snow that we can see on the rooftops and scattered across the grass came the previous night and was melted by the sun and the pressure of cars. On our way out of town, we stopped at McDonald's for breakfast. Mom had her customary Egg McMuffin, while I consumed scrambled eggs and a yogurt parfait, and we discussed that we were headed to the mall. As we resumed our drive and passed a gas station, she said, "*Wow*, has the price of the mall gone way up!"

"What did you say?" I asked.

"I said the price of a mall is really high."

"I'm not sure I understand," I said.

"The price of the mall is high. It's a dollar sixty-five."

"Oh, yes, the price of gas is way up," I agreed. She frequently comments on the price of gas. In fact, almost any time we have passed a gas station since she has been here, she's remarked with surprise on the escalating price of a gallon of gas. We're beginning to see this inability to find the right word in other situations too. Last night, Mom came into our room twice after going to the bathroom. Sue was awakened and said that Mom was more disoriented, verbally, than she's ever seen her. She kept saying things that Sue could not understand.

On our Sunday by ourselves, Mom and I spent five hours together. At the mall, we shopped, walked for exercise, shopped some more, and enjoyed lunch at the food court. Mom ate half of a turkey sub, and we wrapped the rest and then embarked on our return trip home. The ride home, possibly because she was getting tired, was the worst ever for circular conversations. Mom repeatedly noticed and commented on the skyrocketing price of gas. I tried to divert her by saying, "The sky looks like it is clearing," (her favorite subject, usually), but she came right back to the circular conversation that either involved the price of gas or the next four things we will do. I was compelled to keep repeating, "We'll arrive home, nap for an hour, go to Marli's concert, and go out to dinner." Mom enjoys music on the radio, even singing along occasionally, but this failed as a diversion for more than a few minutes at a time.

After Mom napped, the five of us headed across town for Marli's school concert. Mom seemed to enjoy herself, even though we were seated for two hours and fifteen minutes, and she did very well at a lengthy dinner with the four of us plus a friend of Marli's, a friend of Raina's, and the parents of Marli's friend. She often engaged the father of Marli's friend, seated next to her at dinner, in conversation, as she had done earlier in the afternoon with the lady seated next to her during intermission at the concert.

As I write this, I am reflecting again on the pattern I have seen to her circular conversations. Once again I ponder that her questions revolve around what is going to happen next. There was the dialogue with Raina on the plane from Florida, the questioning of me when we drove to Syracuse, the questions as we rode to St. Lawrence University for my class, and now the questions as we drove to and from the mall as examples.

On the positive side, her physical health has been really good the past ten days—not one complaint about stomach pains or headaches, not one request for medication. This is a stark contrast to the constant stream of complaints about aches the first five weeks and constant requests for all kinds of medication. The book Gary sent, *The 36-Hour Day*, indicates that she can be expected to exaggerate discomfort or pain.

Probably, the first five weeks, she was experiencing some discomfort due to increased disorientation caused by the move to Potsdam, and maybe now we have that behind us. It was particularly difficult two weeks ago when she was constipated. We ended up taking her to the doctor, who prescribed an enema, which Ginny applied. That immediately reduced the complaints of pain and the frequency of feeling the need to go to the bathroom, but then came a day of loose movements and insisting that we come into the bathroom to look and inspect her underwear. However, since then the complaints have eased off, at least for much of the past two weeks.

In many respects she acts like a kid—accepts what we tell her but makes requests with a kid's appeal. She often asks if it is all right to eat something, wear a certain garment, or do something—even asks Raina. But if we say, "No, the doctor said you can't have any more medication," or "The doctor says you have to eat more," she usually accepts it.

I am still feeling uncomfortable that I didn't take Mom to Florida so Gary could be with her when Marli, Alice, and I went down in early October, even though Gary and Sue agreed with the decision, and I know it was best for Mom. I reminded Gary that he, Laurie, Todd, Brian, and Sally are welcome to visit any time. Or, I suggested, maybe when we do make the last visit to clean up The Classic apartment, I can bring Mom down with us.

I am convinced that as long as Mom continues to be okay physically—and as long as the nights don't become impossible—we will be able to keep her with us in our Potsdam home and possibly be able to have her travel with us. She now seems to accept being here and recognizes and takes comfort from each of us, even at the times she can't recall our names or where she is.

Monday, November 20

Mom had a rough time staying in her room and finding her way between the bathroom and bedroom between midnight and approximately three this morning. Is it possible that the pace of Sunday led to the restlessness and disorientation in the early morning hours today? It's hard to tell. I'm still searching, without much luck, for cause/effect relationships between her behaviors and what kind of day or night she has. This morning Mom accompanied me to the store to pick up the paper since Ginny will not be here for the three days before Thanksgiving. She asked to have the days off, and since I have no meetings and Susan and the children only have today and tomorrow for school, we said okay. On the five-minute ride to the convenience store, Mom again commented on the high price of gas but found the word "gas" easily this time. At home a few minutes later, she fumbled for words a couple of times. Otherwise it was a pretty average day, which included a few episodes that, while humorous, also highlighted the depth of the dementia that is gradually, yet inexorably, taking hold of her mind.

While the rest of us were sitting around the family room reading the local newspaper, Mom picked up Raina's school folder, with the name RAINA MESIBOV in large letters on the outside. Raina said, "Grandma, that's mine."

Mom said, "No, it's not; it's mine."

"But, Grandma, it has my name on it."

"No, it doesn't. That's my name: Raina Mesibov."

"Grandma, my name is Raina Mesibov."

"No, it's my name."

Finally, Marli intervened. "Grandma, your name is Rhoda, not Raina. They sound alike and both start with the same letter."

"Oh, I didn't know that."

Raina is also in charge of the large chalkboard that we placed in the upstairs hallway, partway between our bedroom and Mom's. It also serves as a barrier so that Mom is less likely to wander into Marli's room. Raina puts daily messages on the board—e.g., "Sue, Marli, and Raina have gone to school. Dad is downstairs. Ginny will be here at 8 am."

I continue contemplating the patterns and lack of patterns in the ways Mom's memory fails her. I e-mailed Gary, and after asking him if he was able to connect with Gail on any of his recent excursions to England, I recalled that he had once told me about an evaluation of a special education student and had pointed out that her mind was like a computer. The fact that she might know something didn't mean that she could recall it when she wanted or needed to. I told him that I am seeing more of this with Mom. You can see the frustration overcome her when she struggles to find a word that she knows is stored somewhere in her memory but which, more and more, she cannot access when she wants to. There are gradual, yet slowly increasing incidents of this kind, as we would expect.

Tuesday, November 21

We will leave for the Thanksgiving holiday tomorrow. Marli and Raina stayed home with their grandmother, while Susan and I visited the Alzheimer's unit of the local assisted living retirement home. We were impressed. It is only twelve miles from our home, and we have heard excellent reports from people who have relatives there. We put Mom on a waiting list, just in case the time arrives when it is needed. When her name comes up, we can decline and still stay on the list. But at least it will reduce the waiting time if and when we need it. I suggested to Gary that he might want to do this with a nursing home in Chapel Hill if he still wants to consider it as an option. Then when he does come here to visit Mom, he can check this one out and compare. I emphasized that there is no rush on any of this—we are just looking way down the road. On the way back from the retirement home, we stopped at the house to pick up Mom, Marli, and Raina, and we all went to a restaurant for lunch. Susan, Marli, and I enjoyed salads; Raina had pasta with marinara sauce; and Mom had a turkey sandwich.

Today, because it is Thanksgiving week and Ginny is off, Mom had a companion provided by the local health care agency from one to four this afternoon. They checked with Tower Administration, and there was no problem with insurance covering it. We'll probably use the companion about three hours every weekend and occasionally for a full day or night—definitely in the near future on a weekend when we have concert tickets in Ottawa. The woman the agency sent is with Mom now and is nice enough, but she is not at all decisive. Along with Mom's indecisiveness, the two make quite a pair:

"Should we?"
"I don't know, should we?"
"What do you think?"
"I don't know, what do you think?"

It makes us appreciate Ginny all the more. But she does seem competent and maybe will get more assertive—or we can, hopefully, help her to be more assertive—with time. Also, I'm not at all sure that we'll have the same person each time since we won't have a regular schedule with the agency; we'll request caregivers on an as-needed basis, on occasional weekends, or if Ginny can't make it on a particular day, as was the case today.

At one point this afternoon, Mom asked, "What's for dinner?" Sue gave a response she almost immediately wished she could take back. "You can finish the turkey sandwich you brought home from the mall on Sunday." Mom quickly responded, "I don't want that; I want something new."

Marli overheard the discussion, saying nothing, but then when Mom asked about dinner again, Marli said, "How about I fix you a turkey sandwich, Grandma?"

"That would be great," Mom agreed.

One thing that is troubling, and different, is that Mom asks to go to the bathroom with increasing frequency. This started a day or two ago, and the requests seem to come almost every twenty minutes now.

Gary e-mailed a "thank you" for my frequent e-mail updates on Mom's condition and confirmed that it sounds like what the book, *The 36-Hour Day*, would have us expect. He thanked me also for the open invitation for any or all of them to visit and suggested that we wait to see what happens with The Classic and a possible Florida visit before making definite plans.

Wednesday, November 22

We traveled downstate to spend Thanksgiving with Sue's mom, two sisters, and their families. Each sister is married with two daughters, and they live ten miles apart. In recent days, Susan and I have discussed our apprehension about this trip. We have learned enough about Alzheimer's to be aware that any change in routine or surroundings can increase the disorientation symptoms of the sufferer. We had experienced this when we brought Mom to Potsdam in early October. She would become more easily agitated and was more easily confused during the first few weeks in Potsdam when contrasted with how she had been in Florida, even with the loss of her husband and all the changes in routine during the month of his hospitalization. But now she has been adjusting to her new routine, the house, the climate, and the people, and we are taking her to an unfamiliar house in yet another new community (new to her, anyway), where she will be surrounded by quite a few people that she doesn't know or knows just barely.

The trip was difficult. Normally it is about five and three-quarter hours plus stops, but it took us more than eight hours. Anticipating a lengthy drive, we left Potsdam around eleven o'clock this morning. Mom needed time to get ready, and I had to stop at the bank and the brokerage office, or we would have left earlier. On the ride down, she continued to ask to go to the bathroom at least once every half hour. Only after we were south of Albany did we get one stretch as long as an hour without a bathroom request.

Thursday, November 23

Thanksgiving dinner was in Chappaqua, at Sue's other sister Cookie's home. and it went extremely well. Even though Mom was a bit more reticent around people she doesn't know than would have been the case a few years ago, she did continue to jump into conversations to the degree her condition allows and the degree to which she found people willing to interact with her. However, she did seem to have more aches and pains and less bright moments than in late October and earlier in November. The frequency of visits to the bathroom continues. While she did, as always, seem to enjoy being around people, how can we assess the effects on her of a different house, new routine, and totally unfamiliar schedule?

Friday, November 24

While the requests to use the bathroom continued, I can see that need is no longer driving them. It is like her requests for medicine when she first arrived in October. They were initially based on headaches or stomachaches (perhaps exaggerated, but with some basis). But after a while, the requests for medicine had become automatic even, I suspect, long after the need had passed. It had taken us about a week of delaying medication—"You just took some, and the doctor said no more until dinnertime"—until we reached the point where she stopped asking.

We're being careful not to deny her use of a bathroom when she needs it, but we are finding it easier to get her to delay a visit for an extra half hour or so.

Saturday, November 25

We drove back today, leaving Briarcliff Manor at eleven thirty, making two lengthy meal stops and several other pit stops, and getting back to Potsdam at nine thirty tonight. Mom was fine on the car ride, engaged us in conversation at times, took frequent brief naps, and had long periods of silence.

Tonight was really difficult. Mom went to bed at ten thirty, with less difficulty than usual. She slept for an hour before her first nocturnal walk. Then she slept another two hours before getting up again, but then she got up at least five times within an hour. At two thirty I found her outside Raina's door, sifting through some clean laundry in the basket that Sue had left there after Raina went to bed. Each time, it was easy to guide her back to her room, pull the covers over her, and have her go back to sleep for a little while—until she ventured back to the laundry basket again.

At five thirty I heard a noise, saw the light on in her room, and went in to find her fully dressed for the day.

I got her back into another nightgown (the one she had been wearing was wet at the bottom), put on clean diaper pants—Depends, which she'd forgotten to put on, although she wears them all the time—and put her back into bed.

Sunday, November 26

I had lots of work to catch up on in my home office, so I didn't have the luxury of sleeping late to catch up on the interrupted sleep I got in the wee hours of the morning. Since this is the end of the holiday weekend, there was no Sunday school, and we were all at home. This morning Sue got Mom to take a bath, but it was a challenge. At one point, Raina described for me the dialogue that occurred.

Sue: "Mom, you need to take a bath."

Mom: "No, I don't."

Sue (using a strategy from the book): "Mom, the water is warm, doesn't it feel good?"

Mom (not moving from outside the bathroom door): "The water is cold."

Sue: "Mom, the water is nice; try it."

Raina informed me, "Grandma really needs a bath; she smells horrible."

Finally Sue succeeded. We had a late breakfast, and Mom seemed cheerful and ready for the day.

There is no question, unfortunately, that more often she is having difficulty finding the word she wishes to use. It continues in evidence all week. She may want to say "food" and instead says "machine," as in, "When are we going to have the machine?" Usually she gets fixated on a word that she has used in another context and then uses that word to mean different things over the next few minutes. This is probably the start of a process where she will eventually lose the ability to communicate. At times it is clear that she wants to say something, but she remains silent in the middle of a sentence as she struggles to find the word. At other times she uses a word confidently, but it makes no sense at all.

Mom has completely stopped asking for or about Aunt Millie or any of her friends. Rae left a message on the machine while we were gone, and I am going to have Mom call her this morning. I want to see if there is any recognition of who Rae is or where she is.

In short, there is some mental deterioration. How much will become more evident as she settles back into the usual routine. We will see what is due to the disorientation of the Thanksgiving holiday trip and how much is just a continuation of the Alzheimer's process. Mom continues to make bathroom visits anywhere from ten minutes to half an hour apart and is in constant need of ointment for the soreness created by the frequency of these visits.

Today the forecast is for freezing rain. We'll have a family day indoors. On Monday Ginny will be back with Mom, and we'll see what Ginny's perception is of Mom's progress or degree of deterioration.

Today was a much more placid day for Mom. She napped for two hours in the afternoon. But the disorientation continues—physical even more than mental—and she is having difficulty wiping herself and keeping sanitary. I'm hoping that she will bounce back in the next few days, but it doesn't look good. On the one hand, as I look back to how she was when we were with her in Florida, there isn't a great deal of deterioration in terms of her mental functions. But the deterioration that is taking place is gradually moving her out of our reach, verbally, and moving her into a position where she is less and less independent. I think of when we were in Florida in late September, and Raina came over to my side of the table at Boston Chicken and said, "I feel like Grandma is slipping away from us."

Because of the physical deterioration combined with the mental dementia, unless there is improvement, we will have to consider bringing in caregivers from the agency to help put her to bed at night. For now we are committed to just using them for a few hours every weekend and for those rare weekdays when Ginny is unavailable. There are bright spots. Mom continues to be cheerful when she doesn't have aches or pains—and even sometimes when she does. She constantly wants to dialogue, and at times, there is a continuous flow of questions.

We watched *My Dog Skip* on tape this afternoon, and it was obvious that she couldn't follow any of it. But when she heard a word or saw a sign, she asked a question.

As soon as I got downstairs to my office, I found the following e-mail from Gary: "We had a wonderful Thanksgiving with the family, and now I am far away in Asia preparing presentations. I survived the trip, but thirty hours on planes is a long time to be en route to Singapore or anywhere for that matter. Glad to hear some positives have returned, but the ongoing deterioration, though inevitable, must be hard to watch. Thanks again for all that you are doing. Will call from Dallas on Sunday, en route home."

I am reflecting on our four-day excursion downstate for Thanksgiving; on Mom's aches, pains, and bathroom visits in the context of what degree the travel and other changes in routine may have affected her; and also I am thinking of the changes brought about for our two girls, Susan, and me since our August visit to Florida. What seems to be weighing most heavily on all of us is the stress of having to always be on guard. It's not any one situation that has been too trying or exhausting; it's the nonstop accumulation of tasks, fears, and uncertainties that is wearying us all. We have to be as much aware of where Mom is and what she is or is not doing at every given moment as was necessary from the time one of our babies reached the developmental stage of mobility—where you could put them down in one spot and no longer be able to count on them being there if you turned your back for even a second. But with a baby, nap time and bedtime and meal times and other routines were much more predictable. Effective use of family members, sitters, and friends could enable one to get more rest, even if insufficient, than we are finding is the situation with Mom.

The stress of caring for Mom is caused by the ongoing sequence of unending needs that Mom generates. When you raise a young child, you have periodic discipline concerns, problems, cuts, bruises, acts of defiance (testing), and even occasional middle-of-the-night visits to an emergency room. But while raising a child, you also have reasonably long periods of stability and opportunities to rotate coverage so that each spouse can grab much needed "space" when the pressure threatens to become unbearable. With Mom in the house, the four of us are on a nonstop cycle of vigilance for her safety, finding ways to occupy her time productively, and addressing all her needs and wants. With a child, your workload gets easier as his or her ability to function independently grows with age, whereas Mom's dependence increases with the passage of time, and her increased dependence on us seems to have accelerated much more rapidly than we had anticipated when comparing November with the preceding month.

Much of our time with Mom is filled with fun, wonderful, enjoyable experiences, as well as the less pleasant tasks, but it all comes together to create the feeling in each of us of being on a nonstop merry-go-round that occasionally feels more like a rollercoaster ride.

Don reminisces about his mother:
I recall a nearly eight-hundred-mile trip from Chapel Hill to Potsdam with Ed in the passenger's seat while I drove, and Mom and Darren (three at the time) were in the back with Darren in his car seat. Mom taught him to sing, "We've 800 miles to go; we'll ride awhile and rest awhile; we've 800 miles to go." Like most children Darren loved repetition, and long after his grandmother would have been grateful to have ended the song, he kept asking how many more miles to Potsdam and then would engage her in yet another verse. Grandma obliged every time.

Todd reminisces about his grandmother:
The time I remember most being with Grandma was driving to Potsdam from our home in Chapel Hill with Grandma and Ed when I was probably around ten. We rarely drove more than two or three hours before taking a break, so an eighteen-hour trip seemed impossible but ended up being lots of fun.

Rapid Deterioration: "I Wish I Could Die"

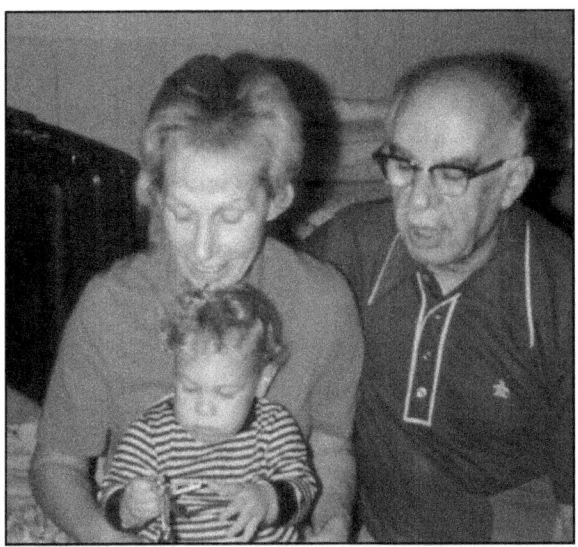

When Darren was a toddler Grandma and Ed drove with him from Chapel Hill to Potsdam singing the same verse over and over and over.

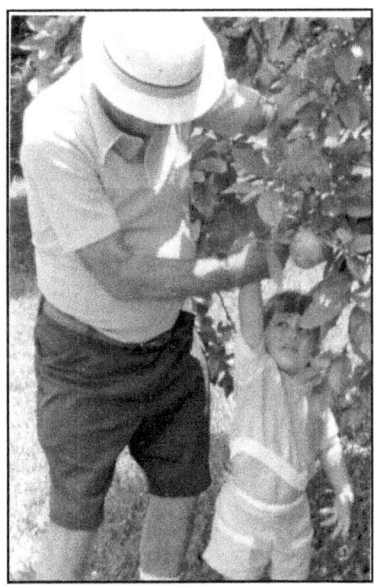

Mom would send Ed into their backyard to help the grandchildren pick grapefruits from their trees. Here he is with Marli, probably in 1987.

Chapter 10

Ten for Dinner

Ten of us lived within a half mile of each other as I grew up; ten of us celebrated holidays together; and ten of us ate meals together when it was convenient. Therefore, it was natural that nine people were the primary influences on my development and certainly had a significant impact on the person my mother became, just as she played a major role in all of our lives. As I think of the people responsible for my genetic makeup and know what I know about Mom's condition, Alzheimer's-related thoughts cross my mind. Would my maternal grandfather have had Alzheimer's if stomach cancer hadn't ended his life at seventy-three? My maternal grandmother's life did end with Alzheimer's when she was eighty-two. The last time I visited her, in a nursing home in 1973, we had to hold the straw to her mouth while she sipped a liquid. She was unable to speak, move very much, or react to anything we said except with a smile. Would my father have had to endure Alzheimer's, or would his father, if heart attacks hadn't claimed their lives shortly after they passed their fiftieth birthdays? Dad's father was stricken two months before my birth.

    The patriarch of our family was my mother's father, Maurice Rubenstein. I loved my grandmother, Fanny, and I respected and liked my father's mother, Ruth (she taught me to play bridge and canasta and baked spice cookies with a delightful aroma that I can still conjure up), but Grandpa was my favorite. We played checkers on the front porch of his home in Lynbrook when I was a youngster. Grandpa was gentle and warm. He had escaped from Russia by boat with the Brody family, and for many years after, both he and my grandmother continued to join his rescuers for an annual reunion. Gail recalls, "Grandpa came over with the Brody family when he was thirteen, and gradually the rest of his family came over. I seem to remember a story about him playing the drums in the Russian army. Grandma, who also emigrated from Russia, was, I think, carried over by her parents when she was three. I have no idea how they met."

Grandpa eventually became foreman of the Adelaar Blouse Factory in the garment section of New York City. He commuted over an hour to and from work almost until his death, most of the time taking the train. I recall that three buses filled with the employees that he had supervised made the trip to a Long Island temple for the funeral services; the image of their arrival has stayed with me, along with an understanding of what that said about his character and his demeanor as a boss.

Although politically Grandpa voted Democratic, as did many Jewish immigrants of his generation, he was generally a conservative individual, perhaps owing to having very little money when he arrived in America and then living through the Depression. Gary tells of how Mom and Aunt Millie would get nervous the infrequent times he would drive to work instead of taking the train. "They thought he was a terrible driver," Gary told me, "because he would drive thirty-five miles per hour, hugging the right lane in a fifty-five-miles-per-hour zone. Then one day he received an award in the mail from AAA for driving fifty years without an accident. Mom and Aunt Millie joked that he may not have had a single accident, but he sure caused a bunch."

There was only one time I ever recalled seeing Grandpa angry, and at that time his anger was directed at me—and I deserved it. I was probably no more than six at the time. Having since become an avid gardener (fanatical may be a more accurate description), I can now understand his rage and inability to conceal it. He was spending the day fishing at Jones Beach. Whether Grandma Fanny initiated it or I asked, I can't be sure, but I ended up picking tomatoes from Grandpa's garden with the instruction, from Grandma, to only pick the ripe ones, "which are the ones that are very red."

After picking the ones that were clearly red, I took a few to Grandma that were pretty red and asked if it was okay to pick them. She said yes, and after that I used my own judgment rather than seeking any more second opinions. In my desire to continue this fun activity, I began to rationalize the acceptability of almost every other tomato in the garden until what anyone else would see as dark green became close enough to red for me to bring it into the house. I don't recall Grandma's reaction when I revealed what I had been doing during the thirty minutes she was probably thinking how nice it was that Donnie was productively occupied, but I do remember Grandpa's verbal rebuke, which was so strong that, as I lay awake in bed that night, I seriously doubted that he would ever speak to me again. He did, and to this day I think of him as such a wonderful role model and loving man.

Fanny was the stereotypical family matriarch of the early- to mid-twentieth century. Family was not just part of her existence; it *was* her existence. I think she only listened to the news, regularly, once in her lifetime, and that was when Gary was of draft age. She listened only to hear if there would be an announcement that the Vietnam War had ended. Grandma rarely traveled or vacationed, and when she came with us to San Francisco for Gary's graduation from Stanford, her only reaction to the beautiful setting and nice weather was, to paraphrase former Vice President Spiro Agnew, "I don't see any difference between this and other cities." Yet she exhibited the delight of a child in an ice cream parlor to be with the whole family and to see her grandson walk across the stage.

Grandma Fanny had sold eggs door-to-door to help Grandpa raise enough money so that they could get married. After that, she was the ultimate homebody. Her passion in life was to cook for the whole family, and as one meal ended, she would ask what we wanted for the next. I can still see her announcing to the nine of us as we cleaned our plates of turkey, sweet potatoes with melted marshmallows, candied carrots, and her special dishes of rice pudding and of macaroni that had been brought to a boil in tomato juice, "Save some room for the roast beef; it will be out in a minute." Gary recalls that her final words to him the last time he visited her in the nursing home were, "Gary, don't forget to put the potatoes in the oven."

One time after dinner—as we sat at the table, too full to want to get up—we passed around a humorous picture. Each of us, in turn, looked at the picture, laughed, and passed it to the next person. When it came to Grandma, she also looked at it and laughed, but something about her reaction made me suspicious and, upon closer scrutiny, I realized she had the picture upside down. She was laughing because she was part of the group, and if the group thought it was funny, it must have been. Years later I saw this same type of behavior characterize Mom's reactions when she was so far along in her battle with Alzheimer's that she couldn't possibly understand what was being said or causing laughter, but she would pick up cues that would let her know how to react. Yes, it could have been at times like these that she didn't want to reveal her lack of understanding, but I think it was more that she wanted to belong to the group. If the group was laughing, she wanted to be laughing and to be seen laughing. Long before Alzheimer's had her in its grip, Mom would react to people, particularly Gary and me, with an affirming nod, laugh, or statement of approval, even at times when she wasn't completely sure why she should, but it was evident that reinforcement was called for.

From the time I left for college until a few years before her death in a nursing home, suffering from Alzheimer's, Grandma Fanny would write to me regularly and always enclose a check for twenty-five dollars without an explanatory note—as if a letter, a stamp, and twenty-five dollars went with any mailing you sent to anyone.

Uncle Kip, the tallest of the ten of us at about six feet (at least until Fred was fully grown at about the same height), was an avid golfer and the comic in the family. In addition to peppering the dinner conversation with jokes and puns, he might disappear for a few minutes and return with a mop over his balding red head to simulate a wig, and he would accompany the visual effect with an appropriate punch line.

As Gail recalls her mother—Mom's sister—Aunt Millie could be persistent and dominating. While we were growing up, she was a terrific aunt, and she and Mom did many things together and were loving sisters. However, Dad may have been glad for the opportunity to move to Maryland once Gary and I were out of the nest since he worried that Mom acceded to Aunt Millie's opinions and subverted her own personality to too great an extent when they were together. Whether it was that Aunt Millie was too intimidating as the older sister or that Mom was too easily intimidated by her is not something I could even guess. I do know that after Mom married Ed and moved to Florida, and after Aunt Millie and Uncle Kip also moved to Florida, there was a ten-year period where the two sisters did not communicate with each other. It may have had to do with Aunt Millie's reaction to Mom's marriage to Ed, but maybe there was more to it. The following two recollections will shine light on each sister's personality:

While I was too young to recall this story from personal knowledge, Aunt Millie had apparently found an expensive coat at a department store that she really liked, and so she purchased it. However, the store had to order it in her size and promised to have the coat shipped to her within two weeks. After three weeks, she called Abraham and Strauss (A&S, as the department store was known) and demanded to know why the coat hadn't arrived. The customer service representative apologized for the delay and assured Aunt Millie that she would locate the coat and see that it was shipped out right away. Another week went by, and no coat arrived, so she called again. This time she raised the level of her complaint to the point where she received even more apologies and an assurance that she would have the coat as soon as it was humanly possible to get it to her. Two days later the coat arrived. The day after that, the same style coat arrived—it was shipped from Macy's Department store, which, Aunt Millie had forgotten, was where she had actually placed the order. Did she return the mistakenly delivered coat to A&S? As too many of us would do, she rationalized that she had earned the extra coat and kept it as a spare.

In 1967, a little over a year after my dad passed away, Aunt Millie and my mother drove to Boston to visit me. I took them to Durgin Park, the legendary restaurant known for prime ribs and cornbread. The waitresses were usually competent, but reveled—in a friendly way—in their reputation for being unsmiling, which had become as much a Durgin Park trademark as the excellent quality of its food. Mom ordered the prime rib special, medium rare, and the rest of us placed our orders. The waitress brought part of our order and placed a side order of french fries in front of Mom. Politely Mom said, "I think I ordered the mashed potatoes." "No, you didn't," snapped the waitress, with a scowl that was not part of the unsmiling "act" of most of the waitresses at Durgin Park. She reached for her note pad as if she wanted to prove she was right. Obviously her own notes indicated that mashed potatoes had been the order because, still scowling and without any acknowledgment, she turned and headed back to the kitchen.

A moment later Mom cut into her prime rib, and it was brown, not the slightest shade of pink or even light brown. "That's terrible," said Aunt Millie, "send it back." "Oh, it's okay; I don't want to bother them," said Mom, perhaps being more accommodating than she should. Aunt Millie would have none of it: "This is one of the finest restaurants in Boston, and Donnie took us here as a special treat. If this is a class restaurant, they will want to know when the food does not come out of the kitchen as ordered." When the waitress returned with the mashed potatoes, Aunt Millie spoke up. "Would you take this back, please? It was ordered to be medium rare."

The waitress responded with a line that was unfathomable, and which motivated me to head for the manager to have a new server assigned. "I can't take it back," she growled, "because you cut into it."

Yes. Millie's assertiveness could be overdone, as with the coat, but it could be a positive quality as exhibited with the prime rib that she insisted be sent back.

Growing up, my brother, two cousins and I were close. Fred, the oldest, was the first to wed and eventually was on his way to a successful career at the University of Wyoming, where he became a revered professor in the political science department until his death from heart failure in 2006.

Fred was two grades and about nineteen months ahead of me. He was by far a better athlete than I, having been named Long Island Player of the Year while starring on the 1957 Nassau County high school championship basketball team and then having gone to Rutgers on a scholarship. The closest I could get to being on a team, despite my love of sports, was to be P.A. announcer at the games. But when we were home together, we loved to play any kind of sport—either just the two of us or the two of us and Gary. We invented games for all seasons. There was the Throwing-Out Game, which was played on the street in front of our houses by two people with a tennis ball, including one with a loud voice (me) who could announce the results. There was Bat Ball, played on the Gillisons' driveway down the block. This required a practice golf ball and a miniature bat, about two feet long, and could be played by as many as four people. Then there was Magazine Ball, which required only a magazine, a Ping-Pong ball, and a chalk outline of a plate drawn on the inside back wall of the garage. Magazine Ball could be played in any kind of weather conditions because the entire game took place inside a closed garage. However, if the family car was in the garage, there was Sock Ball, which was played in an upstairs bedroom with a magazine and a rolled-up pair of socks.

I recall a time when I was twelve and there was a loud noise as the rolled-up socks smashed the light bulb that hung from the center of the bedroom ceiling. Mom came running to the foot of the stairs yelling, "What happened? Is anyone hurt?" "Mom," I yelled back, "we're fine. Gil Hodges just hit a grand slam home run!"

Fred's father, Uncle Kip, was successful. Fred knew that his father wanted him to go into accounting as well, so when Fred graduated college, he went to work for Price Waterhouse. But accounting wasn't for Fred. He could easily have been the character in *The Producers*, played by Matthew Broderick, who sang the song "I Want to Be a Producer," about the humdrum, regimented life of an accountant. After a few years, Fred went back to school to study Russian, which took him on a path through Indiana and Purdue Universities and to the political science department at the University of Wyoming, where he was in the midst of a productive and satisfying career when we exchanged many e-mails during the months that Mom was living with us. Fred had married his high school sweetheart, Carole, in 1962. Carole was a cheerleader the years Fred starred on his high school basketball team, and she was at his side forty-four years later on January 1, 2006 when his heart gave out. Fred authored a number of books during his career, on topics ranging from the mafia to taking responsibility for one's medical decisions, which he wrote following his ordeal undergoing heart surgery when he was in his early forties.

I remember, admiringly, a quote I can paraphrase from one of his books: "When you speak with someone, act as if this person is the only person in the world and give him your complete attention." A student who took a course from Fred and worked closely with him told of how Fred always made him feel special by giving him such undivided attention. He also respected how Fred would give a priority to a phone call from his wife or children, no matter what else he was doing.

Cousin Gail, escaping a failed marriage in the late 1960s, embarked on what was intended to be a brief stay in London and that became a lifelong residency. Within a year she was talking with her new accent as if she had been born in London. It took a little longer, but then came her wonderful family, starting with husband John and then the children, Rachel and Adam, and now Rachel's husband, Jason. Gail continues to enjoy a career in counseling. Years after we were grown, Gail revealed to Gary and me how she suffered as a child from the chauvinism of her brother and two cousins. Of course, by then we were much too old to do anything about it. She said she was continually disappointed that we didn't let her play Magazine Ball, Bat Ball, or any of the other games she wanted to be part of—except if we were unable to find an available male, and only then, if we were absolutely desperate. In our defense, this was before most people gave any thought to equal rights for women, and whenever we entertained the thought of allowing Gail to join us, our first reaction was, "She's a girl."

Gary, younger than Gail by more than three years, adds this remembrance. "I had the same problem of not always being allowed to play with you and Fred because I was too young. But if you needed more people, I was picked over Gail because being younger was not considered as bad as being a girl. I remember the games I was allowed to play with you and Fred, but I don't recall playing ball with Gail. Recently, I asked Gail what we did when we played together. She said we played cowboys and Indians, and we were Roy Rogers and Dale Evans. I asked her why she never seemed to want to talk about that, and she said she didn't want to hurt my feelings because she always wanted to be Roy Rogers, and, as the younger, I was forced to accept being Dale Evans."

In recent years Gail, John, and Adam spent two weeks visiting our home and touring Quebec City with us. Susan, Marli, Raina, and I have visited them in London twice. One of those times was for Rachel's wedding. Gary travels to London on business occasionally, so he and Gail have had far more opportunities to connect firsthand. The four cousins always remained close and, more importantly, always felt a special bond. Fred's passing has caused Gail, Gary, and me to draw still closer and to value our communications and time with each other even more.

Marli reminisces about her grandmother:
Being with Grandma made me feel like I was entering another world. She was very relaxed and always calm. She was comfortable not having a plan for the day or having a plan, if that's what other people wanted. I don't think it was passiveness. I think she just enjoyed either option.

Brian reminisces about his grandmother:
I always looked forward to being with Grandma because she made sure our visits included (and more accurately, were designed around) all kinds of fun activities for Todd and me. And she always had Velamints in the glove compartment of her car.

Ten for Dinner

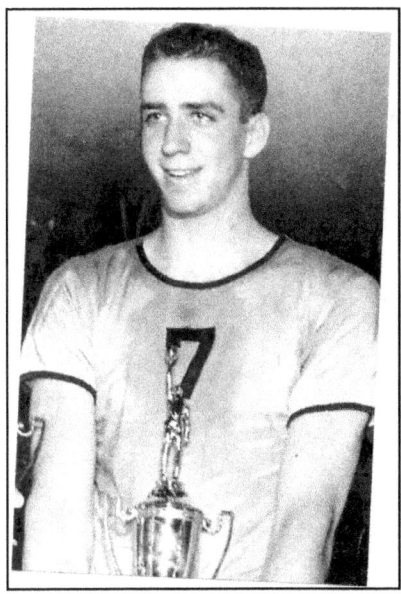

Fred, as a senior at West Hempstead High School, holds the trophy his team won for being county basketball champions in 1957.

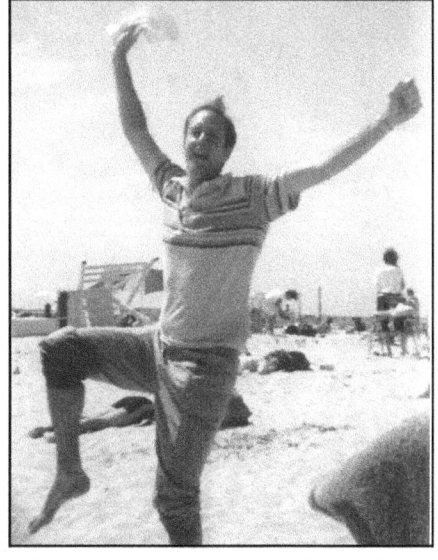

"Fred loved to clown around," according to Carole. Here he is shown doing a *Zorba the Greek* dance on a beach in Crete in 1984. "He used that book and the movie in one of his classes and he really admired the author."

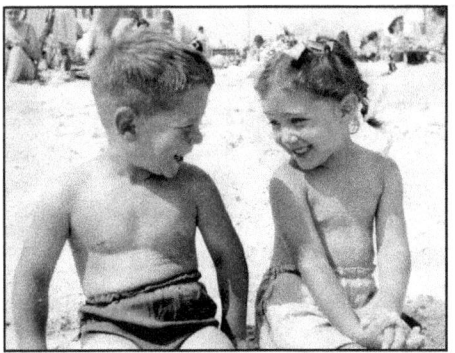

Don and Gail in 1944 (approximate) in a photo the family has always adored. Their mothers often talked about seeking publication in *Life* or *Look* magazine.

Appreciating Mom Through the Lens of Alzheimer's

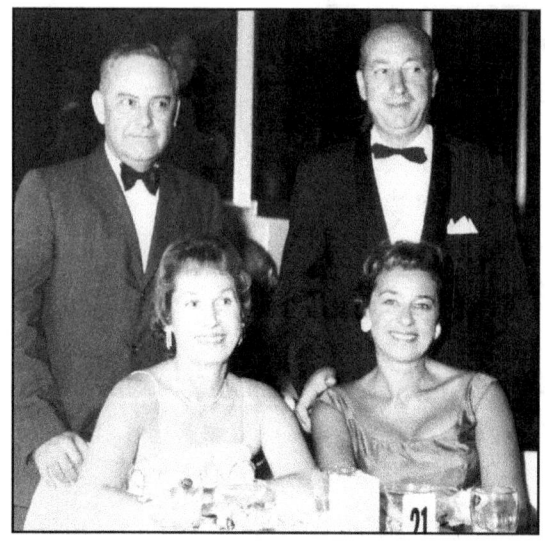

Mom and Dad (left) and Aunt Millie and Uncle Kip.

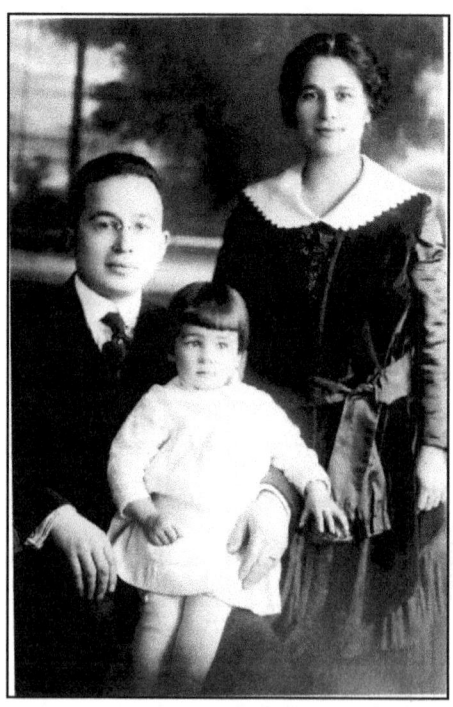

Grandpa Maurice and Grandma Fannie
with Aunt Millie (1916, approximate).

Chapter 11

Mom Falls Four Times

Monday, November 27

When we brought Mom to Potsdam, my thought was to keep her as long as we had the ability to manage her care and, hopefully, as long as she could recognize who we were and benefit from being around family. It was the right decision. For whatever disruptions in family life or challenges it has thrown our way, we are all by far the better for it. The constant reminder of what's important in life, the warmth of having a family of five at meals together (six when Darren is with us), the dialogues, the cooperation among us as we try to do what's best for Mom and to decide how to handle the many challenges posed by her condition have all helped us to mature as individuals and as a family.

It's not always easy. I lose my temper at times; I get frustrated at the lost work time, but it really is all worth it. The girls watched their bathroom get dismantled and got frustrated the first week Mom was here, but they have adjusted. They even take in stride an occasional visit from Mom at one in the morning, when she will walk into one of their rooms, turn on the light, and begin rummaging through a desk drawer looking for only God knows what. Mom thinks that she knows what she is looking for, but she can't articulate it.

Clearly Mom has benefited from the kind of love she's receiving, the frequency of having people around her who care, and the constant challenges to her intellect. The addition of Ginny has been a stroke of good fortune: she has a sunny disposition, loves being with Mom, and handles her beautifully and with a sense of humor. "Rhoda," Ginny will say, "if you keep calling me Sue, I'm going to get out my old bowling shirt with the name Ginny on it and wear it every day."

Since our return from the Thanksgiving trip last Saturday, Mom continues complaining of aches and pains more than usual, but it's nothing substantially out of the ordinary in terms of severity. The frequency of the bathroom visits also continues, although not quite as bad as the two days prior to our trip or the first half of our Thanksgiving visit. When rested, I can handle her with a sense of humor. At three in the morning, when we just returned from downstate, I screamed, pleaded, yelled, and begged her to go back to bed and, "Go to sleep, for God's sake!"

My mind is made up. We will have to start using the caregiver service more frequently—and perhaps evenings for help getting her into bed and to monitor her throughout the night. I am finding it impossible to get my own work done, and it is beginning to drain all of us—mainly because of her increased use of the bathroom (each trip requires us to be vigilant) and the increased frequency of the late-night and early morning sleepless adventures. I am also finding that the same amount of sleep I have been getting by on— five to six hours a night is all I usually need—is no longer enough. Maybe it's because of how strenuous it is taking care of her when I am awake, or maybe because sleep is broken up by the number of times I see or hear her get up to go to the bathroom, or maybe just because I sleep lightly in anticipation of a problem. All I know for certain is that I no longer seem able to get up easily at six o'clock, even if I do get to sleep by midnight and have the potential for six or seven hours of sleep.

Mom's bathroom habits are another major factor. At times she will emerge from the bathroom with her Depends around her knees or ankles. "Let me help you pull those up, Mom." Or she will walk out of the bathroom holding used toilet paper and say, "Look at this," and I will say, "Mom, let's throw this in the toilet." Often she will say, from the bathroom, "Come here, there's something I want to tell you." Then she will show me the inside of her Depends, soiled. I will either say, "That's so small, ignore it and pull up your pants," or, "We'd better put on a clean pair of Depends."

The combination of the difficulties in getting her to bed at night, often lasting until two or three in the morning, and her bathroom habits have led us to conclude that we need more help to keep her here. I suspect that we will need to put her in a home within a few months because the rate of deterioration is reaching the point where, even with outside help, it may be difficult to maintain her here. I am also beginning to wonder if she is nearing the time where she may be so unaware of her surroundings that she won't realize that she is in a nursing home. She accepts wherever she is. While she recognizes us, she is unaware of time. If I walk in the door after being gone for a day, she reacts as if I had been in the room two minutes ago and had just gone to the mailbox.

Tuesday, November 28

This morning Ginny had to attend a funeral, and rather than get a caregiver for just a few hours, I decided to be with Mom and take her to my college class and then to lunch. Ginny planned to return at one forty-five. Also, I thought it may be one of the last times Mom and I could have quality time like this at one of my classes; she had really enjoyed it the last time. I went to wake Mom at eight o'clock and could not get her to move an inch. This is typical in the sense that she has become used to sleeping until nine thirty or ten. She will make bathroom trips every twenty or thirty minutes from bedtime until two or three in the morning, but then she will sleep soundly until around five or six, go to the bathroom one more time, and then conk out for about another four hours.

I just couldn't awaken her. Finally at eight forty-five, I yelled, "You have to get up. We have barely enough time to get dressed, go to McDonald's for breakfast, and make it to my class."

Nothing.

"Mom, do I have to do to you what I would do to one of my campers—pour water on your head?" She smiled and moved a little. Then came extended time in the bathroom. Finally I said, "Mom, unless we leave now, there will be no time for breakfast, and I may get fired from my job if I don't make it to class."

"I'm hurrying, Don, but I'm not done yet."

After several similar conversations, we finally left the house. No time for McDonald's, I ran into a convenience store, grabbed a doughnut and orange juice, and we made it to class at ten. Mom ate half a doughnut and drank her juice, had her five pills, and observed the class quietly. The students ran the whole class, so I sat next to Mom and observed and occasionally commented. By midsemester, my classes are usually a series of student presentations with groups of three or four students each having from twenty minutes to an hour for a presentation they were assigned earlier in the semester. This morning's presentation was on "Multiple Intelligences" since this is a class for future teachers. At 11:05, Mom asked to go to the bathroom (she had been able to make it through the entire class a month earlier), and I took her to a private bathroom across the hall, where I could watch the closed door from the entrance to my class. She was in there for half an hour and came out just before the end of class. As we walked toward the car, she emphasized her need for a bathroom, and I decided to take her right home rather than out for lunch.

On the ride home, Mom occasionally complained of not feeling comfortable. "Something's wrong," she said a couple of times. Later in the day and the next day, she said the same thing. She doesn't say this often, and she doesn't belabor it when she does. And it was no more than she had said fairly frequently the first two weeks she was here, in early October.

Wednesday, November 29

It was around ten thirty this evening. Mom was in the bathroom, and Sue and I were in our room getting ready for bed, correcting papers, and watching TV. We heard a thunderous noise. (Gary might have been able to hear it in Singapore, it sounded so loud.) Sue yelled, "Oh, my God!" and we both ran to the bathroom to find Mom's body draped over the rim of the tub, with her face down in the tub. I pulled her up, and she was groggy either from the fall, the sleeping pill taken an hour earlier, or both, but she said weakly that she was okay. She wasn't holding any part of her body nor acting as if in pain. I walked her back to bed and tucked her in.

As soon as we had Mom settled, I said to Sue, "Please call United Helpers in the morning"—they run the Alzheimer's unit of the home we had visited just before Thanksgiving—"and see if they can expedite the process of accepting her. We have to do something. Mom can't be left unattended at night anymore. I'll call Med Link or Caregivers and see if they can cover us overnight until they have an opening at the home."

For the rest of the night we slept in shifts, and each time Mom's bedroom door opened, one of us ran to the bathroom and made sure that the door remained open so that we could see Mom. As soon as she got up from the toilet, we were there to guide her back to the bedroom. Mom then visited the bathroom about seven times between eleven that night and two. The third time, as I put her into bed, she complained of a pain under her arm. The next time she complained of a pain lower down. Each time she seemed to have a pain somewhere; however, she never complained of the same pain twice. I hope it isn't serious. I decided to wait and see how she feels in the morning. At two o'clock in the morning, she went to the bathroom for the last time tonight, and I guided her back into bed. As I tucked her in, she looked up and asked, "What time is it?" Totally exhausted, I said, "Mom, it's after two." "Oh," she said matter-of-factly, "that's not bad. It could have been a lot later."

Thursday, November 30

Mom was her old self. Ginny found some dried blood on her head, but it seemed more like a scrape or scratch (obviously from the fall) than a gash. Mom showed no other effects from the fall and didn't complain of any soreness or pain. Ginny said that

Mom has not been able to get back to the intellectual level she had maintained a few weeks ago in their game playing, but she did recognize the railroad in one of the games near the end of the day, which apparently, according to Ginny, is a higher-level intellectual plane than she had operated on most of the day.

What had caused the fall in the tub? The upstairs guest-room toilet faces the bathtub, which is about three feet away. At first I assumed that Mom had stumbled from being dazed by the pill or disoriented by the time of night. However, later that night as I watched her get up from the toilet seat, I saw her turn so that her back was to the tub and then try to pull up her Depends. As she turned, she fell backward. I was there to catch her, but otherwise she would have fallen into the tub just as we found her earlier in the night. I am convinced that this is what had happened.

As we had decided yesterday morning, Sue called the doctor to set up an evaluation for entry into the nursing home. Sue described the fall and other symptoms of Wednesday night, and the nurse said, "She may have had a small stroke, and that could have caused her fall. Even the brief feelings of pain later in the night could have been small strokes."

I don't see any evidence of this, particularly in the way Mom acted today, so my theory is still that she slipped as she tried to pull up her Depends. But the stroke theory is possible and might account for her increased disorientation.

Ginny is keeping a daily journal, which she leaves out for us to read so that we can keep abreast of how Mom is doing when we are not home. It is a manila bound notebook with a green border. She records a paragraph or two each day that tells us what she did with Mom and what she observed. Other caregivers occasionally record in this book what happens on their watch as well. Ginny's journal for today reads:

Ginny's Journal:
Up at 8:30 am. As I was washing her hair, I noticed a small cut on her head, probably from her fall in the bathroom last night. Sue made an appoint-

ment for December 13 to have Dr. Kay check her out completely. While Rhoda was eating breakfast, she choked on a piece of toast, then a few minutes later she choked while drinking tea. At about 2 pm, Rhoda was calling out for Don. I told her that Don was at a meeting. Could I help her? Her bottom was sore, so I had her put some Vaseline on it.

As a result of our experiences last night, we converted our main-floor study into a small bedroom for Mom. She will have a half-bathroom directly across a small hallway, fewer than four feet from the door to what is now her new bedroom. There is not much area for her to get in trouble. When she leaves her room at night, there will be almost no place to maneuver except to the bathroom. Once in the bathroom, there is little room between the toilet and the sink for her to fall.

Other than the move to the main floor bedroom, today was a fairly typical day for all of us. If Gary had been at the dinner table, he would not have seen much difference from his last dinner with Mom in September. She was cheerful and often repeated, "I didn't know that," and, "Oh, really?" Clearly she forgets almost everything that is said and can repeat things without fully understanding them. "Ed died, really? When did that happen? Do I have a new husband?"

After dinner we took Mom to the historical museum, where Marli and eleven of her schoolmates were playing music for a one-hour reception. They performed from a second-story balcony while the audience, including us, sat below in a relatively small room. Mom ate a cookie and sat quietly beside me. "Mom, look up there," I said, "It's Marli, the girl with the cello."

"Oh, really, where?"

"Up there."

"Yes, I see her. Who is Marli?"

Yet she seemed to recognize that this is a person in her life. The PTA president came over and began speaking with me. Mom interjected:

"Where does your daughter go to college?"

"Amherst, and she loves it," the PTA president replied, enjoying, as we all do, that someone is taking an interest in hearing about her family. Then she continued to dialogue with me about her daughter and her plans for the future. A few minutes later, Mom interjected again:

"Oh, that sounds very nice. How long has she lived there?"

"About five years."

"That's wonderful," Mom commented.

"Yes, she really likes it."

"How many machines has it been?"

This completely nonplussed the PTA president, who found a reason to move to another part of the room.

After forty-five minutes, Marli completed her musician's role at the open house and was ready to leave. On the plus side, Mom had made it almost an hour before asking for a bathroom. This hasn't happened much the past two weeks. However, as we entered the car, she was in need again she said, notwithstanding having made three visits to the bathroom in the fifteen minutes prior to leaving the house only a little more than an hour ago. We put her off, and she was fine on the ride home.

We arrived back home at eight fifteen and got Mom into her bedtime routine. However, for the first time, she was sleeping downstairs on the main floor. Also, we are now bringing in an all-night caregiver whom we will station in the kitchen within direct eyesight of Mom's new bedroom. Having Mom on the main floor may also make it easier for the caregivers. Except for a morning trip upstairs to bathe her, she and her caregiver can remain on one floor all the time, with access to her new bedroom, bathroom, the kitchen, and the family room.

Mom easily accepted her new quarters and smiled when I said, "You won't even have to walk upstairs except once a day for your bath." She was in bed by nine thirty and had already been up again and into the bathroom twice by ten o'clock when her new all-night caregiver arrived to stay until six in the morning. The caregiver's major responsibility: "When Mom opens the bedroom door, be there to be sure she doesn't fall on her way to the bathroom, help her back into bed after she comes out of the bathroom, make sure she has on dry Depends, and help her pull up her Depends if she forgets."

Friday, December 1

This morning Sue and the kids watched Mom's door from six o'clock, when the Med Link caregiver left, until I took over at seven. At seven thirty Mom walked out of her new bedroom, and I gently turned her around and guided her back into bed. She was completely disoriented, much more than usual, and kept asking me, "Have you gotten the machine yet?"

"No, Mom."

"Well, try to get it now; I'll wait."

"Go to sleep, Mom, and I'll look for the machine while you sleep."

She went back to bed after recycling this discussion a few times. Ten minutes later she was up again—similar routine, just a different topic—went back to bed for another ten minutes, got up—similar routine—and went back to bed again, this time to sleep for a while. Ginny has been here since eight fifteen.

At 9:33 a.m. Ginny yelled down to my basement office, asking if I wanted her to wake Mom. She's apparently been asleep since shortly after 8:00 a.m. Ginny said, "Mom's sound asleep—doesn't stir when I go in." Normally I would ask Ginny to wake Mom so that we can get her on an earlier schedule. But with the Wednesday night fall and the adjustment difficulties yesterday, I told Ginny to let her sleep late this morning. "Let's see if her disorientation is less and her spirits better with a really good night's sleep. Also, with the help of Med Link caregivers tonight and the weekend ahead of us, we can handle a different sleep schedule better than would be the case if it were earlier in the week."

Ginny's Journal:

We did some walking inside; when we reached the kitchen area each time, Rhoda would say how nice the sunshine looked. While walking through the kitchen, Rhoda noticed a box. She read out loud, "P&C Donuts are best." I reminded her that she had eaten half of a P&C muffin, and she said, "Yes, it was VERY good!" Rhoda also noticed some things that were attached to the refrigerator and told me that they were outdated. She is very verbal today, but sometimes it's hard to understand her—she may be trying to speak of something in her past.

What's the status now? Everything is under control. Ginny will continue to come in from seven or eight o'clock each morning (depending on my schedule for the day) until four or five in the afternoon, Monday through Friday. Med Link will supply someone every evening from ten o'clock until six in the morning and will also supply someone for spot shifts on weekend days and early evenings or any other time we need to go somewhere and need coverage. I no longer think it's feasible for us to take Mom with us if we travel much more than forty-five minutes from home. Nor are we any longer able to leave her alone with Raina or Marli, as we have been doing, because of the problems with going to the bathroom and needing someone to actually pull up her Depends or look at them and help her change them. The kids have done much more of this than I would have expected—and without complaint—but the assistance Mom now requires is getting to be more than would be fair to expect of them.

Tower Insurance will cover the Med Link people for about another eight hundred hours, at least two months at our current rate. United Helpers said that Mom is tenth on the list for openings at the home, anywhere from a few weeks' to a few months' wait. Mom has a doctor's appointment this afternoon; originally she was to have her regular monthly appointment next Wednesday. This afternoon's appointment is to evaluate her for United Helpers and also to see if there is further analysis of the cause of her fall.

I sent the following schedule to Med Link, indicating when we will need caregivers:

All nights from 10:00 p.m. until 6:00 a.m.

Weekends from 6:00 a.m. until 10:00 p.m.

On a lighter note, Marli interviewed Grandma for a school project. Her project was to interview an Alzheimer's patient. Sue was present for the first part of the interview.

"Grandma, where were you born?"

"I don't know. Sue, where was I born?"

"Grandma, I want you to answer."

"But Sue knows; I don't know."

"Grandma, when did you meet Harold?"

"I don't know. Don was there, so he would know. Ask him."

"Grandma, Don wasn't born then. He wasn't there."

"Well, if Don wasn't there, then I wasn't there."

Then Raina walked in and she tried to answer all the questions for Grandma. Marli became upset with Raina. Sue intervened and took Raina out of the room and left Marli alone to finish the interview, which Marli welcomed.

Sue said afterward that at times Marli became so hysterical with laughter at Grandma's responses that she had to shut off the tape recorder.

Saturday, December 2

Mom complained of discomfort again today but couldn't identify the cause any more than to say, "I just don't feel right." I called the doctor's office and, fortunately, it is Dr. Kay's weekend to be on call. He concluded that she just needed an enema. *Wow, do I feel stupid.* Now it all makes sense. Mom had been constipated a month ago and had acted much better right after the enema that was applied at that time. I guess I got in a rut of expecting her to exaggerate every ache and pain so that maybe I didn't take it seriously enough when she did complain. Also, you get to expect deterioration—physical and mental—so when something happens, such as an increased number of bathroom visits, you tend to accept it as part of the disease rather than suspect it to be a symptom of a different problem—as you would if anyone else expressed the same complaint.

The good news is that now that I realize that the constant need to go to the bathroom may be just a short-term problem, curable with an enema, her condition doesn't seem quite as dire. I had resigned myself to accepting that the frequency of bathroom visits would continue to get worse. There is still the worsening disorientation; and the fall the other night was real, which indicates the need for around-the-clock supervision to the degree we are now providing. But the possibility that the frequency of bathroom visits may be curable is encouraging and may also lead to more consecutive hours of sleep at night—for Mom and for us. She is still a delight to be with.

Mom had a good morning, despite the discomfort. Her Med Link companion was with her from nine thirty to twelve thirty while I tried to get some work done. Sue and Raina went to temple to set up for tomorrow's bake sale. Marli was in Watertown with the school debate team.

Mom's ability to remember continues to experience good and bad times. The caregiver informed us that Mom had looked at a family portrait and had told her that three of the people are her sons, and two are her daughters. One of the daughters is actually a picture of Mom. On the other hand, another time when the caregiver asked Mom how many sons she has, she immediately said, "Two: Gary and Don."

At twelve thirty, Mom and I went to the university for lunch. Mom expressed some discomfort on the ride over, so I limited her to soup. We were joined at our table by one of my students, and Mom engaged and charmed her as she continued to demonstrate her curiosity, intellect, and humor. When we got home at two, she took a ninety-minute nap. This was highly unusual. I kept expecting her to pop out of her bedroom.

Ginny is an angel. Even though it is a weekend and she is not on duty, she agreed to come over to apply the enema. Ginny had to wake Mom to begin the enema. Then she yelled down to the basement for me to call the doctor because there was an excessive amount of blood in the stool as the enema had its effect. Ginny said there was no blood when she did this a month ago. She did notice a tiny amount of blood in Mom's stool two days ago, and she had called the doctor then. He and Ginny had attributed this to internal hemorrhoids. Obviously the flow this time was more than Ginny was willing to attribute to hemorrhoids.

I called for Dr. Kay, but he was in an emergency situation, so I spoke with another doctor who was on duty for the weekend. He said that there was no emergency as long as she wasn't losing blood at an alarming rate; and she's not. It's not continuous bleeding, just blood coming out as Mom "unconstipates," if there is such a word. He suggested that I call Dr. Kay on Monday morning because the cause does have to be discovered. He said that it could be simply the irritation as Mom ceases to be impacted (or compacted, or whatever). But he said it's conceivable, although not likely, that there could be a cancerous growth causing it.

Sunday, December 3

Darren arrived early in the afternoon from Flagstaff and immediately set to fixing everything around the house for us. He is quite handy—doing it for a living now as he buys fix-it houses, fixes them up himself, and then rents them. Later in the afternoon, Darren, Marli, and Raina were left in charge of Mom for an hour as Sue and I went to the supermarket. When we returned they had quite a tale to tell, and they told it quite matter-of-factly:

Mom rose from a nap, but they saw her headed for the bathroom, so they relaxed. She detoured into the kitchen, pulled down her pants, and leaked on the floor. Marli and Darren stood dumbfounded for a minute before starting to clean up. Raina immediately took charge of Mom and said, "Let's go into your room, Grandma," and proceeded to guide Grandma through a clean-up and clothes-change routine.

Monday, December 4

We finally feel like we have things under control. Mom slept very little Saturday and Sunday evening; she was out of her room frequently, according to the caregiver. But not having to deal with it and being able to get a full night's sleep made a world of difference for Sue and me. The enema also made a world of difference. Mom seems happier, with no complaints of discomfort for the past two days. She's up, around, and inquisitive.

Each morning, it seems, for the past week, following a relatively sleepless night for Mom, Sue has said, "Well, at least she'll finally sleep well tonight." Each day Ginny has limited her naps, and each night she has slept poorly. Finally last night, the report was that Mom was only up once every hour or two. This morning she was up and alert at eight thirty; whereas, for the past few weeks, it was quite an ordeal to get her going in the morning before ten, and even that was difficult.

I e-mailed Gary with an update, and I described the lack of alignment between how much or how little Mom naps during the day and how well she sleeps at night. He wanted to know, "Is there any pattern yet with the sleeping, or does it still seem random?" My response was: "It is somewhat random. If she builds up several days of insufficient sleep, she does tend to do better the next night. A lot, I think, is tied in with her comfort level (e.g., constipation, aches, headaches, whatever). Sometimes we're aware of it, sometimes not. Today was a good day, but at one time she did say that she was uncomfortable. I asked where, but she couldn't tell me. I asked if she had pain; she said no. I asked where she was uncomfortable; she said she was uncomfortable, but she didn't know where.

"I think part of it is just the disease. Even when she is cheerful, rested, and comfortable, she paces unless she is kept busy at an event or in a situation (temple, a play, a meal), where she understands that the expectation is for staying still. It's almost as if her mind is constantly working, unless kept otherwise occupied, and the inability to focus causes a degree of discomfort that requires physical movement. I suspect this may influence sleeping patterns and limit her ability for lengthy sleep except when exhausted. The one pattern that seems to hold is that she will sleep for two to four consecutive hours to conclude her night of sleep—sometimes, as I have described, to the point of not being able to be awakened easily. This doesn't seem to happen during the first two-thirds of her time in bed at night."

Gary, a clinical psychologist, responded, "It is an interesting observation about her mind being constantly working, and that her not being able to focus may be a source of discomfort for her."

Ginny's Journal:

The sun was shining. Rhoda wanted to go outside for a walk, so we bundled up and walked for a little while. It was very windy and cold, but Rhoda enjoyed the outdoors. Rhoda had a good afternoon with a few short naps and then visited with her grandson, Darren. She noticed Darren's two dogs outside and wondered who they belonged to. We did some walking inside, also played Spill and Spell; she wasn't real interested in the game, but played a little and was napping when I left.

Tuesday, December 5
Ginny's Journal:

I left Rhoda alone for one minute when I saw her enter the bathroom and assumed she would be safe in there while I went into the kitchen, but as soon as I disappeared from her sight she must have turned around, walked right back into her bedroom, pulled down her pants, and leaked on the chair. I think when Rhoda reentered her bedroom she probably thought she was in the bathroom and the chair was the toilet.

We have noticed that when Mom emerges from her room—even though the bathroom is only a few feet directly in front of her—she will usually turn left or right and begin searching for the bathroom. This time she apparently turned completely around and returned to her bedroom, thinking it was the bathroom. Maybe she thinks she is still upstairs, where she did have to make a turn to get from her bedroom into the bathroom.

Wednesday, December 6

Mom was in the kitchen with me when Ginny arrived. Ginny fed her a breakfast of cereal, clementines, prune juice, tea, and water and gave her the morning medicines. Mom seemed a little more confused this morning. Twice she told Ginny that she had to go to the bathroom, but upon arriving at the bathroom, she asked Ginny what she wanted her to do. When Ginny asked her if she had to use the bathroom, she said no. Ginny did several exercises with Mom, and Mom did them very well. Ginny told me, "Rhoda didn't recognize herself in a picture this morning. When I had previously asked her who was in the picture, she had always told me that it was her."

Later in the morning, Mom complained to Ginny about the number of pills she has to take. Ginny explained that there are new pills, one is vitamin E and the other a stool softener, and Mom seemed to be okay with this explanation. She napped, and when Ginny first woke her up, she was very argumentative while in the bathroom. She didn't want to sit in order to go to the toilet, but on her next trip a few minutes later, there was no problem. After some exercising they looked at pictures, and Mom was able to recognize herself, Ed, and her grandchildren.

After lunch, she was very tired, and as she lay down, she asked, "How long can I sleep?"

"Five to ten minutes," Ginny teased.

"I'm serious," Mom shot right back.

Ginny asked her, "How long do you want to sleep?"

"About thirty minutes," she said.

I find it interesting that she appeared to recognize that Ginny was not being serious when she said "five to ten minutes," yet she obviously felt that "thirty minutes" was a more realistic response. Does this indicate a degree of critical thinking?

Tonight we are having our first major snowstorm of the winter. There are at least six inches on the ground, with another twelve to fourteen inches possible, according to the forecast. Betty has already called to say that she cannot make it to our house. Darren has volunteered for overnight emergency service. I think he saw Sue and me withering with exhaustion. We put Mom in bed at eight fifteen, and she resurfaced at least ten times between then and ten thirty, sometimes within minutes of the door being closed. Most of the time it was not to go to the bathroom but just to wander aimlessly (at least it appeared to us to be aimlessly) until one of us corralled her and ushered her back to her makeshift bedroom. She came out of her room again, and she asked me to sit and talk with her. She kept saying, "It's not right. Will it be okay tomorrow? It just hasn't been the same."

She's not as articulate as a month ago when she was talking about her confusion and saying that something was wrong, and that she wished she knew what it was. Yet I think she was trying to say the same thing. She was more lucid than usual, and I think she was in one of those moments where she knows something isn't right and struggles with that and is scared by it. I said, "Mom, I'll think about it, and we'll see what we can do in the morning," the same as I will often say when I can't understand what she means. She repeated, "But how can it get better? I don't understand what it is."

I continue trying to compare Mom's behaviors with how she acted when we were with her in Florida in September. Because her mental agility can vary so much from day to day—and even within the course of a day—it is difficult to assess the degree of deterioration. When she says things out of context, can't find the right word, or acts confused, it is sometimes difficult to know if this indicates ongoing deterioration or just a temporary lapse. She had many ups and downs when we were with her in Florida, so it's difficult to know whether, overall, she is sliding back and at what rate. But clearly, the two instances of urinating—in the kitchen and on the bedroom chair—and the total inability to find the bathroom at any time without help, are significant slippages. These would not have happened even a month or two ago. Generally though, yesterday and today have been really good: a lot of nice conversations with Mom.

By eleven, Susan and I were more than ready for sleep. Following through on his offer, Darren substituted for Betty, and he slept on a mattress we positioned right outside Mom's door. He came upstairs and called into our room at about four o'clock in need of a clean nightgown for Mom. Other than that, Sue and I got a good night of sleep, thanks to Darren's willingness to stand guard.

Thursday, December 7

School is closed for a snow day. Ginny couldn't make it in for the day shift, but Raina and Marli were home, so we were okay. Darren awoke at one thirty this afternoon. What a team the three children have formed as they have each given Mom so much love—and have given Susan and me relief from the challenges of caring for her.

The weather improved by noon, so I took Mom and Raina to the bank to cash some checks. We went to the post office and then a small indoor mall in town, where I left them for half an hour so that Raina could give Mom some exercise by walking with her. I also gave Raina two dollars to buy them each a doughnut at the bakery. Part of my purpose was to keep Mom occupied for a couple of hours. Ginny was off because of the storm, and Sue needed time to get some things done around the house. Just keeping up with the laundry Mom generates is a task; she wet the bed last night.

When I went to pick them up, they were still walking. Raina immediately informed me that Mom had four oatmeal cookies but was insisting that she only had one. Mom then proceeded to validate Raina's claim—even though she continued to insist that she had eaten only one cookie—because when we arrived at home she was too full to eat her sandwich. She napped and then ate the sandwich in midafternoon, still insisting she had eaten only one cookie at the mall. But she was cheerful and friendly.

At five thirty Mom awoke from a brief late-afternoon nap and asked, "What's going on?"

At a little past six, Marli and Darren were making fajitas for dinner, and Raina and Mom had been playing dreidel at the kitchen table for twenty minutes. This was significant because it has been becoming increasingly more difficult to engage Mom in an activity and to keep her involved as evidence of further deterioration continues to accumulate. As she prepared for bed, I put toothpaste on her brush for her, and she began to brush her face. I opened my mouth and pointed to my teeth and then guided her hand toward her own teeth before she was able to start brushing.

Friday, December 8

Mom's signature has been getting progressively smaller. It's extremely neat, but absolutely tiny—you need to look really closely to read it. She has been in good spirits the past couple of days. She seems to feel well and is going to the bathroom less, but it is still much more frequently than when she first arrived in Potsdam. She has increasing difficulty locating the word she is looking for and often uses a word spoken by her or someone else a moment ago to try to express something in the next conversation (e.g., "Donnie, when can we meet the cereal?").

The supervising nurse from the caregiving agency came to examine Mom and put a call into Dr. Kay to see if anything could be done about her poor sleeping habits. Without the pills we don't have the risk of grogginess, and I'm not sure how much help the pills have provided anyway. The caregiver is also afraid that lack of sleep could lead to illness.

Several of the caregivers from the agency have indicated to the supervising nurse that they won't accept another assignment here. We (and the nurse) suspect these are caregivers who thought they would have concentrated time to work or read at night and were frustrated by the frequency of Mom's interruptions. The nurse agreed that the caregivers should accept this as part of their job. Some caregivers are willing to come back, and they enjoy Mom. They all agree that Mom's temperament is great. I think part of it is a tight labor market, which makes it difficult for the agencies to be selective in hiring. Also, the head nurse acknowledged that they had been overscheduling some of their caregivers. It is not atypical for a caregiver to arrive here to be with Mom overnight, having already worked many of the previous hours and having to be on duty for much of the next day. The nurse said that they are trying to limit the assignments they give to each of their people. She acknowledged that for a caregiver to be up and down with Mom, for an entire night, could be stressful if the caregiver hasn't had a good day of sleep in advance.

Darren expressed an interest in the Oldsmobile Mom and Ed have owned since the early '90s and maybe some of the furniture. I told him that we are offering the furniture to him, Brian, Todd, or anyone who wants it. I said that I would discuss the car with Uncle Gary and work out a fair price. I am still waiting to hear from Sandra at the Florida brokerage house. I am not happy with her delay in sending us the dates of the purchases of Mom's investments. Larry did say that a trust had been set up by Mom and Ed, and that either Gary or I (he couldn't remember who) would receive a check for $3,750 within a few days, representing the first quarterly payment. Gary and I had agreed that we would direct that right into the new brokerage account in Potsdam with the annuity money and the additional funds from the Florida bank account that Gary is going to send.

I called Gary to let him know that a friend whose mother also has Alzheimer's suggested that he call the IRS and ask them to send him the form that Gary is required to sign in order for the IRS to be able to discuss anything about Mom's taxes (should it become necessary). The friend said that without this form, the IRS will refuse to answer basic questions or to discuss anything about Mom's tax returns. He said that it can take some turnaround time to submit the form and get authorization, and that's why he was suggesting Gary do it sooner rather than later. Once this process is completed, he can call the IRS at any time, and they will discuss any aspect of the tax returns. I told Gary that I would send him all the receipts I have (mostly medical) at the end of the year for forwarding to the accountant.

Gary thanked me for this information and said that Darren should take whatever he wants from the Florida apartment because he doesn't think that Brian and Sally have room for more furniture; Todd and Katie are about to move again, so they are not in a position to take anything. He added, "With regard to the car, I think that is like the other things, as far as I am concerned, so I don't think Darren should have to buy it if he wants it."

Monday, December 11
  Ginny's Journal:
  Rhoda got up at seven fifteen just wanting to walk. I offered her water or juice, but she didn't want anything; I showed her the deer outside by the swing set, and she was "amazed!" We did some walking and played a game. It took a long time for Rhoda to figure it out today—but finally she made some words. She's in a good mood today. We recently discontinued the sleeping pills entirely, and there have been no noticeable setbacks in Rhoda's sleeping habits.

Tuesday, December 12
I woke at six and walked Frisky, our fifty-pound mutt—part Terrier and, as Susan likes to say, part Heinz (meaning fifty-seven varieties). Then I had my high-fiber breakfast cereal and was in my basement office working at seven while Sue stayed on the ground floor in case Mom woke up before the next caregiver arrived. Sue is home because of a furnace problem at her school. The night caregiver left at seven, and Ginny is off today; a new caregiver, Billie, came in at nine thirty, which relieved Sue from keeping watch for Mom. She was still sleeping, probably due to taking the sleeping pill for the first time in a while. Sue called for me to come up at nine forty-five. She said that Billie had tried unsuccessfully to awaken Mom. According to Sue, "Billie reached for Mom's pulse, and I got really scared." Mom then got up but, according to Sue, was extremely disoriented, not making any sense. Sue said that Billie had taken Mom upstairs to give her a shower. A moment later Billie came down to the main floor and said to Sue and me, "I'm worried; she's complaining of a pain in her arm, and she's stooped over the toilet as she sits."

I raced upstairs as Sue yelled, "Might be a heart attack," and went for the phone. When I got upstairs, Mom was starting to stand up from the toilet and was pulling her Depends up over her knees. She looked up and smiled. I said, "Good morning." She responded, "Good morning." Then she looked past me and said to Billie, "And good morning to you."

I said, "Do you know who I am?"

"You're Don." Then she looked past me and asked, "And who are you?"

"I'm Billie. Do you have any pain?"

"No, should I?"

"Does your arm hurt?" Billie asked.

"No, does yours?"

I joined them for breakfast a few minutes later, after Mom finished her shower.

I expect that it will be a normal day, hopefully even better than the past two weeks now that Mom has had her enema. Helen Lobell called while Mom was in the shower. She was going out for the day, but Mom could call her tomorrow morning.

Wednesday, December 13
Ginny's Journal:

It was eight fifteen when I arrived, and Rhoda is up. Don got her dressed, and she is eating breakfast. After, while brushing her teeth, she complained of pain in the left shoulder blade near the bra area. I put some Bengay on her back, and she says it feels better. Down on the couch for about five minutes, then needed to get right up to go somewhere, but not sure where, and then Darren came into the room, and she wanted to ask him some questions. Not sure of her questions, but she needed some answers. Darren said, "Maybe we should ask Don when he returns." Down to couch for rest at 11:17 am. I woke her at noon to get ready for Don to take us to lunch at Giorgies Restaurant. Rhoda was happy to have Darren accompany us to lunch and told him so. In car ride to and from, she was very talkative.

Early this afternoon, a lady came to give her an evaluation that is required to make her eligible for an opening at the home in Canton, if and when one should arise.

"When were you born, Mrs. Meister?"
"Don, when was I born?"
"Do you know how old you are, Mrs. Meister?"
"Don, how old would I be?"
"Mrs. Meister, do you know what year you were born?"
"No, I'm not sure?"
"It says here 1917."
"Oh my, that long ago—can you believe it?"

Isn't it interesting that she doesn't know the answers to any of these questions, yet she does recognize that 1917 was a long time ago?

Several times between two and three this afternoon, Mom asked to lie down. "I'm very tired." At three thirty we left for the doctor's office. From then on she was a different, more vibrant person. Dr. Kay said that she is in good physical condition, and that he does not think that she has suffered any strokes. He took a urine sample and will have it tested for a urinary tract infection, but he said that she was constipated. He suggested yet another enema because he said she is "packed," and that may account for the frequent trips to the bathroom. I did notice that the bowel movement last night was not as loose as it has been. Maybe that was part of the problem, once again, which accounts for her still frequent visits to the bathroom.

Mom has put on a pound since her last visit (back up to a hundred). This is significant because the doctor is worried about possible weight loss as the disease progresses. She had a good dinner, went right to bed at eight thirty (without a pill), and was sleeping at ten o'clock when the caregiver arrived.

Thursday, December 14

The caregiver said that Mom only got up about four times during the night to go to the bathroom—less than usual. She told us that between three and five o'clock Mom awoke several times, opened her door, peered out, and then went back to bed without leaving her room.

Friday, December 15

Ginny's Journal:

Went outside for a walk, which Rhoda enjoyed. Nice and sunny with temperature at twenty-two degrees. I asked Rhoda how she liked winter in New York. She replied, "Pretty rough." I said, "Kinda cool," and she replied, "Yeah, a lot cool!" In early afternoon after some naps, she came into the kitchen and was talking to Darren. She was talking to him and me like we hadn't seen her in weeks. Quite a normal conversation except for her perception that it had been a long time since she had spoken with Darren. She napped for fifteen minutes at 2:12 pm, and when she awoke she wanted to see Raina. Ate grapefruit, walked, visited with Raina, and down to nap at 3:50 pm. Up at 4:20, played game with Raina and me.

Saturday, December 16

With Mom on the main floor and needing constant vigilance, we now have close to twenty-four-hour coverage, and it has turned me into a bean counter, or at least I feel that way. Maybe I've inherited some of Mom's genes for bookkeeping, although I am not as thorough as she would have been. The caregivers we hire through an agency are paid by the insurance company, and I don't have to get involved with that. But I pay the caregivers hired privately by us on the last day of their weekly shifts, which can be any day between Thursday and Sunday. Several have requested to be paid in cash—not to avoid taxes since they know we are reporting what we pay them to the IRS, but because they work so many daytime hours that they have difficulty getting into the village while their bank is open.

I have gotten into a routine that might be humorous if it weren't also expensive. Every few weeks I go to the bank and withdraw between $3,500 and $4,000, and I keep it in an envelope in the second drawer of my dresser. Sometime during the last day of the week that a particular caregiver is working, I bring the cash downstairs to that person, usually while the caregiver is sitting with Mom and playing a game, watching TV, or feeding her or while Mom is napping. I like this system because it limits the times I have to go to the bank, and I know the caregivers appreciate receiving their pay weekly and in cash.

Monday, December 18
Ginny's Journal:

Rhoda was up at 8:40 am, and seemed very confused. She didn't seem to be able to follow directions like, "Take your socks and slippers off." Also, didn't know what "wash your face" means. She said a lot of mixed-up words, for example, "They were sentence." They made no sense whatsoever. She took out rollers and clips to do her hair, combed her hair, and put the rollers back in the drawer as though she had used them, but she hadn't. I started down the stairs with her, and Rhoda said, "Are we going to the cemetery now?"

Tuesday, December 19
Ginny's Journal:

Rhoda seemed in a good mood today—much better oriented. Before her bath, she put her rollers in her hair. This is something she had been doing in the past but not lately. We sat at the kitchen table visiting and talking about the snow coming down. Then we walked into the family room and looked at the Jewish calendar and then some holiday cards on the mantel above the fireplace and some more that are on the piano. We sat on the couch, and Rhoda began petting Puffball, the cat. They both enjoyed that until Rhoda drifted off to sleep.

Wednesday, December 20
Ginny's Journal:
Very confused today. We played Scrabble. Rhoda was unable to comprehend at all. We played the dreidel game, and she enjoyed that. "I WON!" as she exclaimed. We played Spill and Spell; she was able to make some words.

Tuesday, December 26
Ginny's Journal:
Rhoda's very interested in family pictures today. She knew some of the people, and, at times, she knows herself and Ed. Also, she picked up the letter that Raina wrote to "Gram" and read it over and over. I put on clean Depends twice.

The year is almost over and I am reflecting on how much more aware we are of the prevalence of Alzheimer's sufferers in the world. As my mother's condition becomes known among friends, relatives and even casual acquaintances, they share their stories and it seems as though everyone has a close relative or knows of someone with Alzheimer's.

It's enough of a challenge for us. How do people manage without the support system we are fortunate to have? How do people address the sufferer's needs and their own if they don't have insurance coverage and don't have enough of an income to bring in caregivers, on an as-needed basis, as we are able to do?

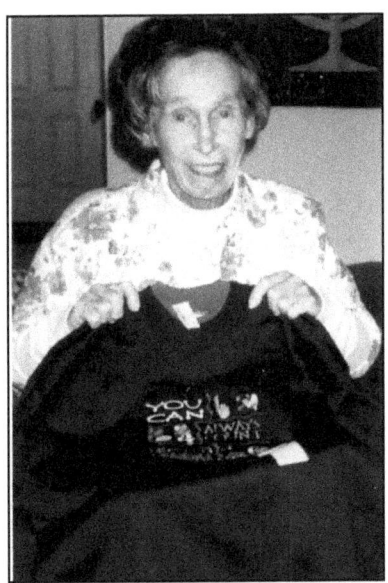

Chanukah at the Mesibov's in 2000 began on December 21 and ended December 29. Mom displays a gift she received from the family.

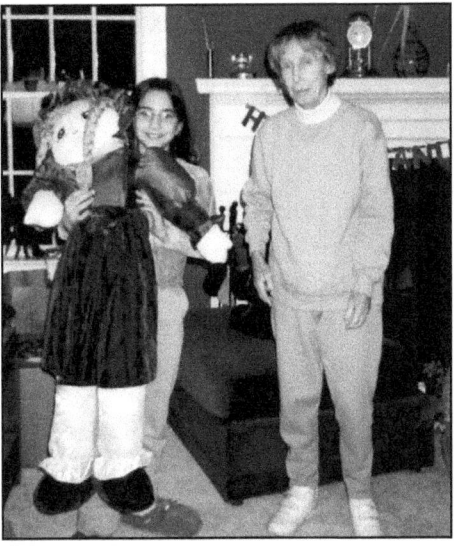

Also, during Chanukah, Raina holds up a large doll, a gift from her grandmother, which Mom picked out with some assistance from Don.

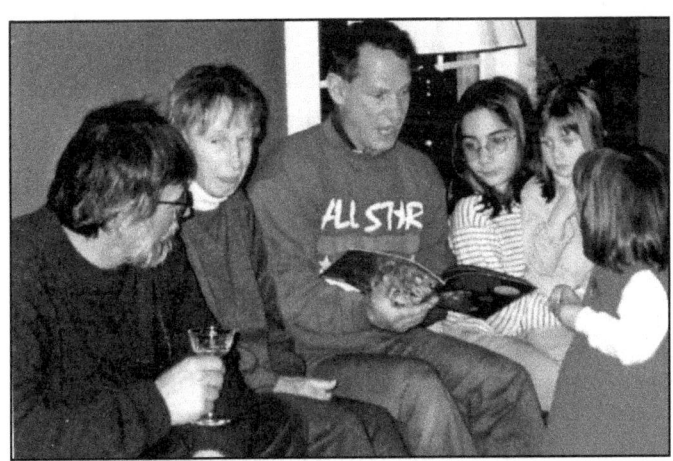

In the living room, friends help Mom celebrate Chanukah with Don and Raina closest to Mom.

Monday, January 1, 2001

We held our annual open house on New Year's Day, an event Susan started years before we met. People stopped by throughout the day, about fifty in all, and Mom enjoyed the gaiety.

Fred sent an e-mail saying, "Tomorrow I get sworn in as a member of the city council, and I think it is the first official meeting. How's it going with Aunt Rhoda? Happy New Year!!!"

Tuesday, January 2

The start of a new year is cause for reflection, and as I think back to Thanksgiving, it seems as though the deterioration of Mom's physical and mental faculties has accelerated from the rate it was happening from the time we first spent time with her in late August until late November. The loss of Ed, the move to Potsdam, and the need to experience a complete change of routines and surroundings could understandably cause disorientation and confusion, even in an otherwise healthy and normal individual. So why does Mom appear to be going downhill more rapidly since mid-November than was the case prior to that time?

Wednesday, January 3
Ginny's Journal:

Rhoda was up at 7:55 am. Her bedding was soaked, as were her gown and Depends. She was somewhat reluctant to take a bath this a.m. and tried to put on clothes instead, but I reminded her how good a bath feels; she agreed. A little confused getting in for bath. Rhoda is very unsteady this a.m. She needs assistance while walking and seems quite shaky while eating breakfast. Getting up from the table, she still needs assistance with walking. Very tired. After lunch she took a fifty-two-minute nap, then we looked at a picture album, and Rhoda had a cookie.

Friday, January 5

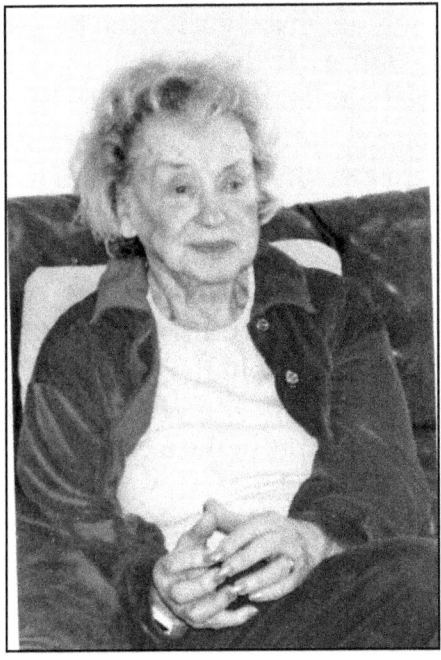

Mom's sister Millie, older by three years, shown in September, 2000. Millie was showing the same early signs of Alzheimer's that Mom had displayed a few years earlier.

From the sounds of recent e-mails from Fred and Gail, I am even more convinced that Aunt Millie is experiencing the same symptoms that we first noticed in my mother. I wrote to my cousins: "While Ed had indicated that it is possible to have loss of memory without having Alzheimer's, your mother seems to be heading down the same path as my mother, but hopefully it is not the same thing." I added that "Your aunt Rhoda is deteriorating rapidly. She has lost the ability to comprehend all but the most simple statements and requests. She often uses one word when meaning another; she cannot connect words with their true meaning, whether she is trying to communicate or trying to understand us or participate in discussions. Most bowel control is gone. The upside is that she now can sleep through the night and has been much more comfortable physically for the past few weeks. It's easier for her to stay with us at the table, do her exercises, and do some things that had eluded her for a while."

While there are improvements in how comfortable Mom is, with the help of enemas, there are downsides to her condition. There are occasional messes to clean up; she has to be treated and protected as you would a baby in diapers; and she can't communicate her physical needs—whether to urinate, BM, go to bed, take a walk, or whatever. There are brief moments when she seems to understand more and to be living in the present. "Let's go for a ride." However, for the most part, she understands as a toddler does. She can laugh at slapstick like a pie in the face on TV or someone falling down, and she seems to understand—or feel—that this is humorous without a cue from others laughing (whether on a soundtrack or someone in the room with her). But she can't process meaning and can't retain a thought for more than a few seconds.

She continues to be sweet and loving and responds to warmth, having us around, being in a room with people talking, and laughing. Raina has really taken her under her wing. At any time you may see Mom and Raina in the living room doing jumping jacks, then marching ("Power walk, Grandma, no slouching") through the living room, into the kitchen, into the dining room, through the halls, and back again.

Tonight for the first time, we noticed another problem. I came in late and joined the family midway through a homemade meal of what we call Matchbox Meatloaf with spaghetti and salad. Growing up, Susan would not eat the meatloaf her mother made, no matter how many recipes Ruth tried—and Ruth did experiment with many different ways to prepare meatloaf. One day her father brought home a pack of matches he'd picked up on the train during his daily commute to New York City, and on the back of the matches was a recipe for meatloaf. Ruth worked from the new recipe a few days later; Susan loved it; and Susan has made us Matchbox Meatloaf ever since we met.

As I sat down at the table, I could see a plate full of meatloaf, spaghetti, and salad in front of Mom on her place mat. Recently Mom's appetite has been pretty good. However, arriving late and hungry, I focused on downing my own food, and periodically I glanced over to Mom. Each time it seemed that her plate looked different, but not much diminished, and yet I knew that she had not added a second portion of anything. Sue and Raina left for Raina's basketball practice, and Marli then pointed out that Mom keeps rearranging her food in neat and different piles on her plate, but is not eating. I said, "Mom, eat some food." She said okay and proceeded to move a slice of meatloaf from one side of the plate to another. It became apparent to Marli and me that Mom did not understand the word "eat," although she did understand that I was asking her to do something with what was on her plate, so she moved food around, hoping that was what I was requesting her to do. Finally Marli took a forkful of meatloaf off of Mom's plate, lifted it to Mom's mouth, and fed her. For the rest of the meal, Marli fed Mom some food, then Mom got the idea and fed herself for a while; then she forgot, and Marli fed her again.

As if Mom's condition weren't generating enough causes for concern, we have been alerted by a caregiver that because of Mom's bowel problems, she should not be allowed to lie perfectly still for more than two hours at a time. That could lead to other concerns. Through it all Mom keeps smiling and showing interest in what is being said, and she tries to join in the conversations even though she is usually completely unintelligible: "Why did you say you are relocating in the exit notch machine?"

We are enjoying the limited time we have with her; all of us have grown immensely through the experience. We exhibit some of the classic symptoms—as a family and as individuals—that books indicate we should expect to feel: frustration (a thirty-six-hour day), anger, wonder, exasperation, and overwhelmed. But we always find a way to get that occasional good night's sleep or those three minutes away for a silent reflection, and then we are ready to dive back in.

I won't deny that Sue and I now fight over the chance to go to the supermarket or to be the one to chauffeur the girls to a practice because the moments alone in the car on the ride back to the house are to be savored for the reflection, peace, and quiet. And I suspect that there are times the kids jump for the chance to run to their rooms to do homework as an escape into a past existence. But when we add up the pluses and minuses of caring for Mom in her current condition, I think we would all say the ups far exceed the downs. What we are each getting—individually and as a family—far exceeds what we are giving or losing (if anything). And even when we are at our worst, it is good experience for us and a good reminder of what is important in life.

Sunday, January 7

Rae called, and we had a nice conversation. I put Mom on, and I first had to show her where to hold the phone; it took a good forty-five seconds for her to figure it out, with my assistance. Then she said, "Hello, Don." I said, "No, Mom, it's Rae." For five minutes, Mom kept recycling the same two thoughts:

"Oh, Rae, are you coming to the plan? What are you doing about the plan? What's that, Don?"

"It's Rae, Mom," I interjected.

"What about the plan? What are you doing about the plan, Don? Yes, but what about the plan? What's happening to the plan?"

After five minutes, I heard her say, "Oh, good, you got the plan."

I got back on with Rae. We spoke for a little while. Rae was fine. I hadn't realized the degree to which Rae had gone through the same thing with Lenny.

Monday, January 8

The events of the week of January 8 to 15 change the prognosis for Mom and explain a lot about Mom's accelerated deterioration of the past few months, even taking into account her Alzheimer's.

Ginny's Journal:
Wet sheet and Depends. Took Rhoda upstairs to bath and assisted with face wash. Rhoda was sitting on the top of the toilet seat while I was running the bath water and somehow slipped off the seat. Hit her head on the wall. I kept talking to her, and she answered me. I applied cold water to the bump on the right side of her head above the right ear. Came down to kitchen, applied ice to her head, called Sue, then Dr. Kay's office, and spoke to the nurse. The nurse said unless Rhoda acts abnormal, she should be just fine. Got Rhoda dressed; she brushed her teeth, had cup of tea, water, two chewy calcium pills. Very verbal, but still confused with sentences. She talked about going to the cemetery. We did exercises, and she continued to follow me and stayed right with the routine. As we visited during the day, sometimes the conversation was okay; other times, just mixed-up sentences.

Tuesday, January 9
Desiree began her shift at ten o'clock Monday evening and finished at eight this morning, when Ginny came in to take over. Mom was up at six, after sleeping through for eight hours, and Desiree noticed that she tended to lean to the right side and drag her right leg slightly. She also appeared "very lethargic" to Desiree. However, by the time Ginny arrived at eight, Mom, according to Ginny, "is raring to go." Ginny took her upstairs to shower, and Mom wanted the shower cap on. She washed her face without assistance and then showered with much prompting and assistance from Ginny.

At breakfast she had a hard time swallowing the large calcium pill. She was quite verbal, and she really enjoyed the sunshine today. She enjoyed going outside with Ginny, even though it was crisp and cold. Even though Mom had assistance while walking today, she slipped and fell to the floor twice. Neither time did she appear to be hurt, but the lack of special circumstances when she falls is frightening because it emphasizes how closely she needs to be monitored and how little independence of movement she retains. Mom spent the remainder of the day quietly and uneventfully.

She is having difficulty eating solids, so we have been keeping her on a nutritious liquid diet. She is so much frailer looking than even a few weeks ago. But today she had such a wonderful smile. Every time I glanced over at her, that smile was as bright as I've ever seen it. She sits so calmly and quietly now, rarely speaking unless spoken to, but so happy and cheerful looking. It's as if she's completely at peace with herself and awaiting whatever will come, but she's so happy in the present, even "as she slips away" (to quote Raina).

I can't envision Mom being with us much longer, certainly not more than a year—maybe only days or weeks. Her rate of weight loss and now the continuing physical decline seem so final. And yet it is so much easier to take because of how she is reacting. I can't say that it will be a blessing for her or for us when it happens. She continues to seem to enjoy every moment, even though it is hard to see what could be enjoyable for her. I guess this is her legacy. Maybe she's hanging around just long enough for all of us to fully appreciate what we've had in her.

Wednesday, January 10

When Desiree arrived at ten o'clock Tuesday night, Mom was in her nightgown and was up writing. At three o'clock Desiree heard a thump and found Mom on the floor. She had fallen out of bed. Mom had slight redness on her right cheekbone and was leaning badly to her right side. Desiree took her to the bathroom and changed her Depends and then put her back to bed. Then she woke us to let us know that Mom had fallen out of bed, was all right, and that she wanted to put chairs up against three sides of the bed (the fourth side is against the wall). However, even though she felt this was necessary, Desiree had the notion that this would constitute "imprisonment," which isn't within the province of the caregiver to do. Susan went downstairs with her, surveyed the situation, and told Desiree, "I can make the decision to put the chairs up, so that's what we'll do."

Desiree is one of our better caregivers. She's about thirty, taking courses at college while she works this job, and has aspirations of becoming a doctor. She's very bright, always offering to bring catalogs with suggested devices that may help Mom, but she has some definite ideas, such as the concept of imprisonment. Raina likes Desiree best, maybe because she talks and plays with Raina and brings her books. Anyway, Desiree is now working for us anywhere from three to seven nights a week.

The quality of caregivers varies greatly. Fortunately, the best of them are on duty most of the time, but that's because we have personally selected the private caregivers whom we have hired. We have requested the agency caregiver, Desiree, who comes most often. As the amount of the available insurance dwindles, we use the agencies' caregivers only on weekends and Wednesdays. We originally located Desiree through the Med Link agency. Since we've cut way back on use of agency caregivers, Desiree often comes four nights a week as a private hire of ours, and then she is assigned by Med Link on Saturday nights. She is excellent. The difference between Desiree, Betty, Shirley, and Ginny, on the one hand, and some of the other caregivers assigned by Med Link is that Ginny and the other three talk with Mom all the time, keep her moving, and love being with her. This is true of some, but certainly not all, of the ones provided by the agencies.

As an example: one of the caregivers an agency sends is sweet, but she loves to talk with us more than to talk to Mom, when we are around. If we are not in the same room, she prefers to watch television, sitting next to Mom, whether it's what is best for Mom or not. Happily, Raina and Marli often pick up the slack. Raina loves to go to the piano and lead Mom in a sing-along. Marli sometimes just sings to Mom as she practices for her public presentations with the school choir.

We've probably seen at least a dozen different agency caregivers. Three or four of them are really good, and we request them as often as possible when we want to be covered by insurance and, therefore, cannot utilize our local caregivers. We've just added weekday shifts from five to ten in the evening, and the caregiver who came last night seemed like a novice—quite shy and unassertive.

Ginny arrived at eight this morning, and it took thirty minutes of coaxing before she was able to help Mom out of bed. She seemed sore from her fall off the toilet seat Monday and her falls yesterday. Mom was very weak today and continued to complain of right-side discomfort. Ginny decided not to take her upstairs for a bath, so she got her dressed and gave her a breakfast of two poached eggs, prune juice, water, tea, and her pills, which include two chewy calcium and one chewy vitamin. Mom had difficulty feeding herself because of a lack of coordination bringing the spoon to and from her mouth. Toward the end of the meal, she was doing better feeding herself; however, the right hand and arm were not working well.

Ginny and Sue took her to Dr. Kay's office, and I briefly joined them in the waiting room on my way to a meeting. Mom looked even frailer than usual; her right eye was not as open as the left, and she continued to lean to her right. She was quieter than usual and sat still, but with a wan smile on her face. Ginny said that she had been like this much of the morning after sleeping late. As I left the three of them in Dr. Kay's waiting room to go to a meeting, I kissed Mom and said good-bye. She looked up with a smile, and displaying more energy than at any time earlier today, she asked, "Where are you going?" This is more typical of Mom but is a behavior that hadn't been evident all day. We all brightened a little. I left Mom with Sue and Ginny.

When Dr. Kay checked Mom over, he confirmed that she probably had a stroke. In fact, he thought she may have had a series of small strokes, and that these may have caused the falls rather than the falls contributing to a deteriorating condition. The result of all these falls is one bad bruise, but no apparent pain or injury. He said that her right arm is okay. What is apparently happening is that her legs are giving out from under her. At first I thought some of her falls when she was in a standing position had been "slips," and we just had to be more careful with her. But yesterday, apparently as she was standing, she would suddenly lose the support of her legs. It's miraculous that she hasn't been hurt. We all now stay close by when she stands, and the caregivers have adapted. Dr. Kay commented on the decline in verbal speech and in her lessening compliance with verbal instructions. He scheduled an MRI for Saturday and prescribed one coated aspirin per day to limit the potential for further strokes.

Thursday, January 11

Mom slept most of the night and much of today. Ginny was concerned about her lack of eating and her frequent choking as she tries to down nearly fourteen pills (the requirement each day, including vitamins). She called Dr. Kay, and he told her to stop all medications, at least until he can assess the results of the MRI. He suggested certain nutritious liquids to give her.

I was gone today from eight thirty this morning until ten fifteen tonight. The caregiving agency sent someone for the monthly health checkup. Mom is okay, except her weight is down to ninety-two pounds—from ninety-nine when the doctor weighed her in October, and a hundred in mid-December.

When I arrived home, Mom was sitting on the couch next to Desiree, thumbing through a magazine, or at least appearing to look at some of the pages. Often Mom and her caregiver will sit on the couch in the family room, which is only about ten feet from the driveway entrance to the house, and this is the only entrance we keep shoveled in the winter. Sitting on the couch, Mom only needs to turn slightly to see someone entering, or she can look straight ahead and see clearly into the kitchen about twenty feet away. As the girls come home from school or I return to the house, Mom and the caregiver are the first ones we see, and they see us as soon as we open the door. This proximity to the kitchen also enables Sue, Mom, and the caregiver to converse whenever Sue is home. At times, the caregiver has to prop Mom up on the couch to keep her from sliding off to one side. Mom now needs to be helped when she walks.

Darren reminisces about his grandmother:
I remember being with Grandma and eating ice cream in front of Morgan's Ice Cream Stand in Potsdam when I was roughly nine or ten years old. Grandma smiled at me as I used my napkin to plug a knothole in our picnic table. I didn't know why she was smiling at the time, but it's clear to me now, as an adult, that she was simply smiling because she enjoyed watching her grandchildren as they grew. Grandpa looked at what I was doing and informed me that it was simply not practical. But Grandma simply enjoyed watching me; she was appreciating, not judging.

Brian reminisces about his grandmother:
Being with Grandma made me feel special.

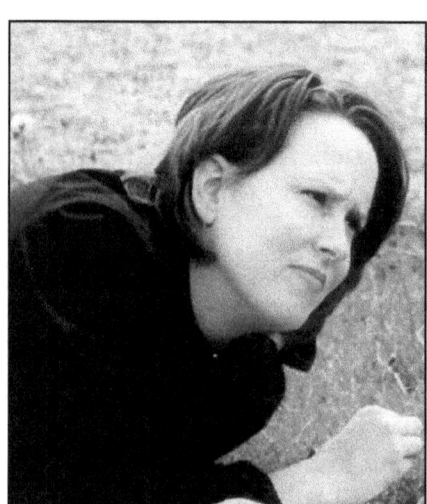

Sally Mesibov, mother of Mom's first great-grandchild, Anna.

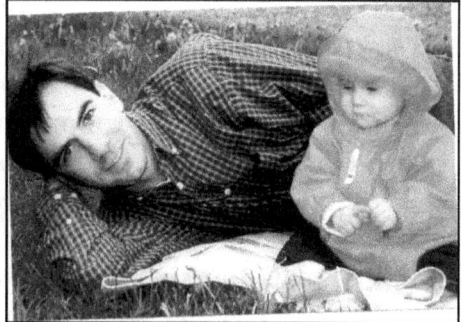

Sally's husband Brian with Anna.

Chapter 12

Mom's Life Gives the Universe Meaning

Friday, January 12

Since moving to the main floor, Mom now sleeps on the top part of a trundle bed. Last night we put her in bed, then pulled up the underneath bed alongside her. This makes the surface of the bed twice as large and, along with the chairs on three sides, there should be no way she can fall off.

Mom woke up a little after eight o'clock, and she had a good sleep. She looked much better this morning. She is not the person Gary saw a few months ago and will never again be. She can only occasionally make sense with the words she speaks, and she speaks less often than even a week or two ago. This past week has definitely taken its toll. But she does not appear to have any discomfort. As recently as four days ago, Sue could place a dozen envelopes in front of Mom, and Mom might take half an hour, but she could arrange and rearrange them in piles. She also could do an effective job folding laundry and sorting things. These activities appear behind us now.

The biggest changes I have seen since October are in Marli and Raina, but probably Susan and I have made the same adjustments. While they have both been exceptionally good with Mom since she first came to live here, there were adjustments we all had to make because of the changes it was causing in our living habits. Both children, understandably, were alarmed when Mom would use their toothbrushes or switch things from one drawer to another. They had some difficulty accepting that things we previously could leave out in the open had to be closeted. Both were particularly annoyed the first times, in October, that Mom walked into their rooms while they were asleep at three in the morning and turned on the overhead light.

I realize now that, at some point, all of these concerns ceased. Everyone now focuses on how we can help. In fact, I recall Gary's comments on the irony of Ed, being a doctor, getting so frustrated with Mom's behaviors that he couldn't look at it clinically and accept it as the actions of a person with a disease. We understood and accepted his frustrations, and we realized that—most of the time—he probably did realize and accept what was happening. Similarly, we as a family now have completely accepted Mom as she is and are able to react to her as you would to someone who has a problem that is not of their own making and that is not within their power to control. In fact, I am probably the least effective, even though most of the time I handle it pretty well. But when I am tired and pressing to get work done against a deadline, I can fall into the Ed syndrome and expect rational responses from Mom when I implore her to "please get into bed so I can get some sleep too." In fairness, Ed had to care for Mom by himself. We have each other to share the responsibility.

Sue is and has been the best at keeping things in perspective. We have both had moments when, in exhaustion, frustration, or exasperation, we have screamed about not having enough time to fulfill our minimum commitments on the job, take care of the children, maintain the house, and deal with Mom's situation. But fortunately, we've usually experienced these bouts separately, and the other has been able to provide a more balanced perspective. However, I realized just yesterday, reflecting as I drove two hours from a workshop I conducted in Ausable Valley, that all of us have learned to keep things in perspective more of the time and to keep reminding ourselves that it is Mom who is enduring the ordeal.

When I see Mom sitting on the couch and that big, broad smile emerges, it gives meaning to the universe. And if she isn't smiling, a few words of encouragement or a joke (whether she understands it or not) brings the smile back to her face. Last night Raina asked me if we would put Grandma in a nursing home, and if so, when. She was lobbying for keeping her here as long as possible. Marli has been like a nurse, feeding Grandma when necessary, alerting us when something has to be done. Both girls have not only learned not to argue when Grandma gives a ridiculous response to something (Raina, that's a four, not a flower) but to smile and say, "You really think so, Grandma?" We are all supporting Mom (Grandma) in the same ways we help each other—and in the same way that she always helped us when we were ill or had a problem. We do everything we can, to the degree possible, to be helpful. The fact that this is a more serious situation than any of us has ever encountered seems to justify a greater commitment of time and effort from each of us.

As I think back to when we first brought Mom to Potsdam, it is clear now that we each had different thoughts running through our minds. Raina was excited, probably because, as Sue analyzed, Mom could become the younger sister that Raina hasn't had. But there is more to it than that. Marli is not only the older sister, but school learning always came easier to her, and so did high grades. Raina shares Marli's level of intelligence, but in school, she doesn't always work to her potential. As a student, Raina is more like I was and like her brother too—bored and challenged to do only as well as she felt she needed to do in order to keep her parents and teachers off her back. Marli, by contrast, seems to enjoy school and rarely has to be policed to start and complete assignments. However, when it comes to caring for Mom, Raina matches all of us with her efforts and successes; and Mom's responses to Raina's attentiveness are as validating as a high grade in school and, for Raina, more fun to obtain.

Marli has confessed that she was not eager to have Mom come to live with us. It was not for any lack of love; in fact, just the opposite: it was because of how much she loved her grandmother. She cherished the memories of her times with Grandma, and she wanted to remember her as she had been. She didn't know if she could regard her grandmother, ravaged with dementia, as the person she had known and loved. To her credit, the support for her grandmother and the love for her that radiates from Marli are not the slightest amount less than what the rest of us offer.

Darren, at age twenty-five, has demonstrated more maturity than I probably would have at that age. He never questioned the decision to bring Mom here. He immediately offered whatever help we would need, and he follows through with frequent trips to Florida and Potsdam more often than we have a right to expect, considering that he has a busy work schedule and life of his own.

For Susan the decision to bring Mom here when Ed passed away was a no-brainer. Obviously we never could have made the offer to bring Mom here if she hadn't suggested it. To me it was a given that even suggesting it to Sue (since it is my mother and her mother-in-law) would place her in an unfair position. However, when Ed became critically ill, Sue was the one who said we had to bring Mom to Potsdam if he didn't pull through. I think Sue underestimated even more than I how much would be involved in caring for Mom. She seems in no way sorry that we've brought Mom here—in fact, I can see that she is happy that Mom is with us and proud of her role in bringing her here—but clearly we had no way of anticipating what the thirty-six-hour day would be like. Through this entire period, Sue has continually faced situations that she couldn't have anticipated, but she rolls with it and just moves to the next level of support for Mom as each week passes and as the support required increases.

Actually, Sue had first proposed bringing Mom and Ed here to live years before Mom's dementia became apparent. Why? In Susan's own words, "We had wanted them to sell their house for several years as had Gary and Laurie. If he was going to move, ideally Ed wanted to be near family so Mom would have visitors when he was gone. But if Ed and Mom were to move, Ed preferred it be to North Carolina because the climate in summer is better than Florida, and it is not too cold in the winter. Gary and Laurie did explore retirement homes in Chapel Hill and couldn't find one suitable within what Ed considered to be his budget.

"Ed also wanted independence, and so I thought if we could put an addition of a main floor master bedroom and bathroom suite and a sunroom so he could enjoy the sun in the long winters, we could have meals together and the house would be big enough for us to all have our own space. But as I said, climate conditions eliminated Potsdam from consideration at that time, regardless of all else."

Obviously, when Ed died and Mom's mind was being destroyed by Alzheimer's, it was a totally different situation. Susan's reasoning for bringing Mom to Potsdam at that time was simple: "She couldn't live alone. It was evident that she was lost. I believe that families take care of each other not just with money, but by providing comfort, being together, and being there for each other, and no one was in a better position to step up to the plate for Mom. I didn't want our children to think that it was okay to do one bit less than was possible for a close family member. I wanted to do what was right in my opinion. I wanted our children, who grew up so far from their extended families, to have, in some way, the experience we had as children."

Did Susan ever have second thoughts as we discovered how daunting the task of taking care of Mom would be? "I always felt that we could make it work. It was good in the beginning and gradually became more difficult as the number of caregivers increased. When we finally decided to consider placing her in the assisted living home, we planned on visiting daily if that should come to pass."

For me, also, the decision was simple. We were positioned to have at least one of the four of us with Mom almost all of the twenty-four hours in a day. And emotionally, I wanted to spend as much time with her as possible—perhaps partly out of guilt that I hadn't valued my father more while he was alive, but mostly, I think, because I was significantly older than I had been when Dad died. I had had so many more years to grow close to Mom and to value her in light of my own experiences as a parent.

From the time Mom and Ed sold their house in Hempstead and moved to Florida permanently in the mid-1970s, they would spend significant portions of their summers up north. For several years in the late 1970s and early 1980s, we rented a condominium near Okemo Mountain in Vermont, and Gary and Laurie and their children would join us for a week.

After Susan and I were married in 1983, we would rent a house or apartment for Mom and Ed in Potsdam, and they would spend between six and ten weeks each summer living within a few miles of us and spending most days in our home. Mom would spend a lot of time with the children, and Ed would read and sometimes relax or even nap outside by the pool under a wide-brim hat and with a fly swatter in his hand. Often we would take day trips or two- and three-day excursions to Ottawa or Montreal, both within a two-hour drive, and sometimes Quebec City or Toronto, each a little more than four hours away. I wish I had been able to spend as much time with my father, as an adult, as I had been able to with my mother.

I had a late-evening meeting with four of my students, and when I returned home at ten o'clock, Mom was sitting on the couch, watching a movie with Sue and Marli. The mail was on the kitchen table, and there was a check from Larry that I will have to deposit in the brokerage account. Mom was unable to endorse it. She has lost the ability to write legibly. When I asked her to sign her name and guided her pen to sign the check, she wrote "Prat" in tiny letters. I signed the check with my power of attorney.

Gary called in response to my e-mail describing Mom's falls. He said that he does not remember in the book we have that falling is part of the problem. On the other hand, he said, The Classic has asked him about that several times, so he assumes that it must be something they look for.

Mom is scheduled to have an MRI done tomorrow, but the doctor thinks she's better off at home until then rather than forcing her to cope with disorientation in a hospital room. Flowers arrived from the Fitzgeralds today, and they are beautiful. A warm and encouraging note was enclosed.

Raina reminisces about her grandmother:
I remember most being with Grandma when she was living with us during those last few months and we would spend every day together after school.

Todd reminisces about his grandmother:
I was always excited to see her.

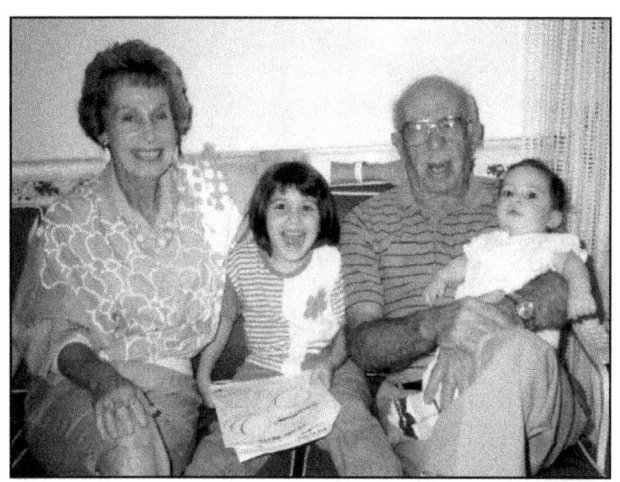

Mom, Marli, Ed, and Raina in early 1991.

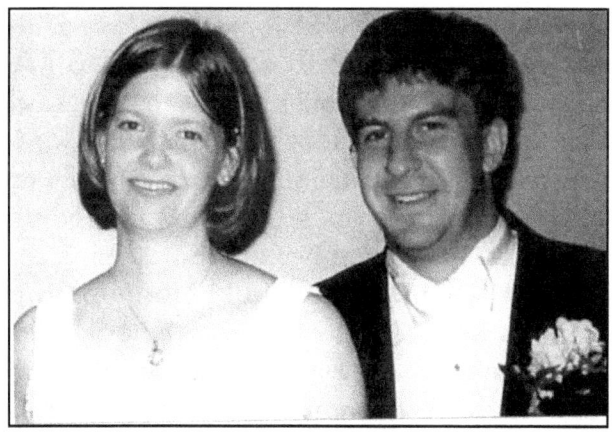

Gary's and Laurie's son Todd and wife Katie; they were married May 26, 2001. Don, Susan, Marli, and Raina didn't know if they could leave Mom long enough to attend the wedding.

Chapter 13

A New Diagnosis: Four Weeks to Live

Saturday, January 13

Mom slept most of the morning and early afternoon; I have resigned myself to the fact that she may never again be capable of more than half an hour of staying awake and being alert. At 1:45 p.m., she was sleeping, having awakened briefly a few times since the previous night. She looked drawn and pale, could barely utter even inaudible phrases, and just sat staring blankly ahead, pretty much even when she was awake. The MRI was scheduled for two thirty, and we hoped to learn if the falls earlier in the week were definitely caused by strokes, as Dr. Kay suspects.

Abby, a new caregiver, had a real chore to wake Mom. It required the two of us to maneuver Mom the short distance to the car; she could not walk on her own. Fortunately, while Abby was on her first case for Med Link, she had previously worked nine years in a retirement home. She knows what she is doing, which is not the case for all of the caregivers that Med Link sends us. She is confident, and she knew how to hold Mom upright to prevent her from falling as we moved from the couch—where she spends most of her time now—to the outside door and then into the car.

At the hospital, Abby went in for a wheelchair and brought it to the car. Mom looked wan and lethargic. We put her into the chair, and she went back to sleep as we wheeled her into the waiting room. Abby sat next to her while I registered Mom and then sat down with them to wait. Abby told me that Mom had six ounces of prune juice early in the morning but had no solids and had refused even water or any other liquid since then. She said she was worried about dehydration. Mom looked really bad. After waiting in an unusually crowded emergency room (unusually crowded for Potsdam), half an hour later than the 2:30 pm time scheduled for the MRI, I wheeled Mom over to the registration desk and asked if I could check her into the emergency room for a doctor to look at her. The receptionist said that we should go for the MRI and then come back and go to triage if we want her to be seen by a doctor.

At three fifteen someone finally came to take us to another room, took Mom away for twenty-five minutes, and then brought her back to us. We wheeled her back to the emergency room, went to triage, and checked her in. Then we wheeled her back to the waiting room and waited until a doctor was ready to see her.

Miraculously, Mom started to come alive. Within twenty minutes she was alert, smiling, laughing at my jokes (as only a mother can do), and responding to our comments. Her words were slurred and spoken with less volume than in the past; I think she clearly has had a stroke. But the color returned to her face; she was wide-awake, and we started wondering why we were even waiting for a doctor. I asked a nurse if we could take Mom home and try to feed her and just bring her back later if there was a problem.

On the ten-minute ride back to the house, Mom again sat in the passenger seat next to me, while Abby sat in the back. I had a new Tony Bennett CD playing, and as he began to sing "White Christmas," Abby said to Mom, "Oh, do you like Christmas music too? I love it." Mom looked at me and asked, "Do we?" She was back to being herself. By four fifteen we were in the house, and Mom ate a full container of yogurt, some soup, and other foods. She even fed herself with her right hand. Mom stayed up until almost midnight, according to Desiree, who took over for Abby at ten. She thumbed through a magazine—without reading anything, I'm sure—and watched TV with Raina and, occasionally, Marli.

Sunday, January 14

Mom woke up a bit groggy and remained that way for a while, but by ten o'clock she was the way she had been at the end of our hospital stay and for the remainder of the previous day—alert and eating. We left Mom with the caregiver, and the four of us went to Ottawa, returned at nine thirty that night, and the caregiver told us that Mom had been alert all day.

I wrote to Gary that Mom is nothing like when he saw her last or even when they last spoke on the phone. She can barely speak audibly, and when she does, it is rarely with words that anyone can understand; in fact, a phone conversation is probably not realistic anymore, except that she can listen. But for the past two days she has seemed completely comfortable and, once again, glad to be with everyone, accepting her condition and the environment as if it were normal. Sue, too, thinks that she might have had a stroke since the right side is the side that seems to be affected, and she's now eating with her left hand. But clearly her speech is still affected, and her energy level has been affected for some time. Abby refers to a "day–night syndrome" and speculates that Mom may have just reversed her sleeping/awake habits. This may be the reason that she has been sleeping past noon and having difficulty sleeping at night. But it was only for a couple of days that we saw this pattern, and now Mom seems to be back on an evening sleep and daytime awake pattern. Nevertheless, whenever Mom gets lethargic during the day, Abby speculates about her syndrome theory. I think Abby is basing her conclusions on too little evidence, like the person who said, "All six-toed cats walk single file, at least the one I saw did."

Raina is having a ball. She likes to be with the caregiver and Mom when Sue and I are either upstairs or out of the house. When Abby first arrived as a new caregiver, we felt a need to alert her—in Raina's presence—that she was the boss, not Raina. We praised Raina for often being correct in knowing Mom's routine but had to remind her, in front of the caregiver, that she could offer advice and suggestions, but it is the caregiver who makes the decisions. In fairness to Raina, she has bailed us out a few times when we have been sent a really incompetent caregiver. Fortunately, on one occasion when we were out at the time, Raina noticed that a caregiver was not giving Mom the required morning pills. She proceeded to tell her which pills to give Mom and also the entire morning routine that she was supposed to put Mom through.

Monday, January 15

At around two thirty this afternoon, I walked into the house after taking Frisky for a walk. Sue was on the telephone, but she whispered that she was speaking with Dr. Kay, and "They've discovered malignant tumors in Mom's brain." When she got off the phone, she explained that Dr. Kay said it probably originated elsewhere in the body, which would mean that she has cancer in other places too. There is a 10 percent chance that it is treatable with a combination of chemotherapy, radiation, and steroids. Dr. Kay wanted to know if we want to put her in the hospital so neurologists and others can check and so that a more targeted MRI can be done on the body, which might enable us to get her back to the way she was a few months ago. Obviously, no treatment can reverse the Alzheimer's.

I tried to call Gary; Laurie was in, and I explained the situation to her. Laurie raised some good questions: Can they give her an MRI at the hospital and evaluate it without her having to stay there? Will the hospital be the best place for her, even for a short time? Laurie emphasized that she would not get involved in making the decision. She was just *looking* at the process. I reached Gary at work, put him on speakerphone, and Sue and I filled him in on the details of her conversation with Dr. Kay.

"Would it have started in the brain?" Gary asked.

"No," Sue said, "the other way around." Sue also explained why Mom would have to stay in the hospital for them to do the tests rather than move her from here to there and back, possibly a few times. "They want to do much more than just an MRI, and it might include intravenous feeding." I filled Gary in on a little more of the background, and we both came to the conclusion that we should put her in the hospital for the few days required and at least get an assessment before we decide on the next step. "Mom doesn't want to live without any quality of life, but this doesn't commit us to anything other than learning the nature of the problem, does it?" he asked.

I confirmed and agreed. We also agreed that I should contact the local hospice and find out what services are available.

Tuesday, January 16

We took Mom to the hospital this morning. When we arrived, Ginny went in and got a wheelchair and then brought it outside, where I had the car as close to the emergency room entrance as possible. Once inside, we checked in at the registration desk. Just as the receptionist was typing the last bit of information into the computer, a scrawny teenager with braces and bright red hair came by and said to the receptionist, "I'll take her from here." He started to wheel Mom toward the long corridor leading to the elevators.

"Which room will we find her in when we're finished registering her?" I asked.

"She'll be on the first floor," the young aide said politely.

"Which room?" I asked.

"You can ask at the nurses' station."

Just then the receptionist interrupted, "I have her listed in room 205."

"That's not what they told me," replied the aide. "They said first floor."

"It says here room 205. Wait a minute," continued the receptionist. "What name do you have for the patient?"

"Helen Chapman," responded the aide. This hardly instilled confidence in us, although we have been at this hospital many times and have always received first-class treatment.

Just before we left, the nurses on duty on Mom's floor assured us that they would watch her closely, and then they put her in a room at the end of the hall, out of sight of the nurses' station. This made us nervous, but we trusted.

Wednesday, January 17

We arrived at the hospital at the start of visiting hours at ten o'clock this morning, and we learned that Mom had fallen out of bed the night before. After this the nurses noted the instructions from the doctor, which had been there all along, to put her in a room visible from the nurses' station. Now they moved her.

Thursday, January 18

Once again we arrived at ten. We found out that Mom was so groggy and in such a deep sleep earlier this morning that the physical therapist and nutritionist—who were sent by the doctor to see how physically fit she is and how much she can be expected to exercise and to swallow—had to reschedule their appointments because they couldn't wake her. Then we learned the reason that they were having trouble waking her was because the nurses gave her sleeping pills Wednesday night to keep her from trying to get up and falling out of bed. Probably, before they gave her pills, she had been getting out of bed and then falling, even though the rails were up.

We instructed the nurses not to give Mom sleeping pills tonight. In fairness, they probably didn't want to use restraints but couldn't watch her closely enough to prevent her excursions. Fortunately she was not hurt by the falls at the hospital Tuesday and has only a big bruise on her side to show for them.

Ginny spent every day with Mom in the hospital. Between her and the nurses, who are excellent, Mom gets four or five walks a day. Ginny and the nurses also came up with a strategy to keep Mom busy and, therefore, less likely to try to get out of bed and risk falling again. The nurses brought Mom a basket filled with crumpled old clothes and rags and asked Mom to fold them. Mom became fully engaged in this activity, got some exercise for her hands, and enjoyed herself. Periodically, when Mom thought everything was neatly folded, a nurse came in, took the basket away, and returned a little later with some more folding to be done.

Saturday, January 20

We came to the hospital to take Mom home. The doctor gave us medication to continue to reduce the swelling in the brain and a pain-killer if she should need it. He also helped us fill out the "No Resuscitate" forms, both for the hospital and for the home in the event that the rescue squad gets called in. We were told to expect a call within a few days to inform us of the results of the MRI and the tests. Mom was asleep in a chair next to the bed in her hospital room when we walked in; we were able to wake her easily, and before long Marli had her engaged in sing-alongs that continued on the entire ride home. Mom smiled as we sang along and joined in occasionally with the lyrics to "Old MacDonald," "Marie," and "Harvest Moon." We arrived home and, perhaps because she was aware that the ability to enjoy Grandma may be measured in days, Marli spent half the day talking with her, laughing with her, singing with her, feeding her, and tending to her. In fact when Barbara from hospice stopped by, she commented on how unusually good Marli was with Grandma. "Better than many caregivers," she told us.

Today went well. Mom seemed to be on a plateau—able to laugh and speak, sometimes she could be understood and sometimes not, but certainly she was able to communicate. She appeared to have no discomfort.

With Marli, Raina, Sue, and the caregivers staying on her to eat, Mom continued to rely on liquid Ensure, drank fluids, and ate applesauce and other healthy foods. I'm hoping we can keep her in her current condition until Gary is able to come for another visit because she really is enjoyable to be around. It's indescribable what she has done and continues to do for us.

We called Aunt Millie, who indicated that she hasn't been calling because she realizes that Mom can't communicate with her. She asked if there was anything she could do and whether she should come to visit. Sue told her it was very cold here, and Millie said that she didn't have appropriate clothes. We told her we would keep her posted. I called Rae while Mom was napping, and we were both in tears by the end of the conversation. "I feel so badly for my friend," she said. Rae said she would call back tomorrow or within a few days to speak with Mom. She did speak with Marli, and Marli said that she and Rae were also crying by the end of the call.

Later in the day, Marli called the Fitzgeralds, and Leilani spoke briefly with Mom. Also, Toby, Laurie's sister in San Francisco who continues to send a card a week, called to see how Mom was doing. Laurie and Toby's father, Dr. Stanley Levenson, called while we were out and left a message on the machine. Then he called again, and I spoke with him. It was good to hear from him. He has always been there for us. Dr. Levenson is a leading burn specialist

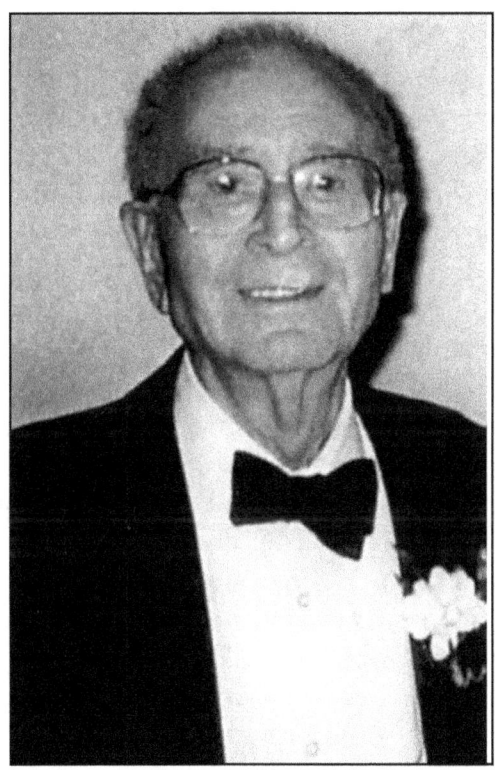

Dr. Levenson was "a master of surgical science who used his expertise to develop the burn center at Jacobi Medical Center in New York into a renowned center of excellence," according to a letter from a representative of the Center, February 3, 2014, announcing that "The Burn Intensive Care Unit will formally be named for Dr. Stanley M. Levenson."

and professor emeritus at the Albert Einstein College of Medicine in Bronx, NY. Whenever anyone in our family or a friend has a major health concern, we contact Dr. Levenson, and he is always gracious and attentive. When he recommends someone to see, he tells us, "I will have contacted him, but be sure to remind him that I am the one who suggested that you see him."

Sunday, January 21

Mom looked about the same today. She appeared a little tired, probably because she slept sporadically last night. She would sleep, then watch TV with the caregiver, then sleep. So today she alternated between being up and cheerful and taking long naps.

I went upstairs to the kitchen from my home office when Sue yelled to me that the hospice lady, Barbara, was here and needed my signature on some papers. She asked if I had any questions. I said that with our state of exhaustion and millions of tasks, as well as worrying about Mom, I was not in a position to read fine print, and I needed to know if anything I was required to sign was significant. She said that it was all standard. She asked if I had additional questions. I told her we needed to be alerted to services hospice could provide that we might need but might not know to ask about. Hospice services will start tomorrow. Nancy, the manager who visited with me in the hospital when I first indicated that I wanted to learn about hospice, will come by personally. Working with hospice, we will have a wider choice of caregivers from whom we can select, and some of the cost will be offset.

Barbara suggested that we contact a funeral home to arrange for transportation to Florida in preparation for the time that it becomes necessary. I called Gary, relayed what I had learned, and let him know that I didn't want to contact a funeral home up here until he had spoken with the Florida funeral home since they will make the arrangements. They may have certain requirements or advice. Ed had prepaid for all funeral arrangements with the Levitt-Weinstein funeral home in West Palm Beach.

Monday, January 22

Ginny's Journal:
Up at 8 am; she seems a little weak, but walked upstairs with full assistance. I had to lift her up for standing position, but then she was able to step out of the tub—she probably had forgotten the routine since she was in the hospital for five or six days. After lunch we did some walking with assistance. She's kind of weak. Nancy Fletcher, RN for hospice, came for a visit today; she took Rhoda's BP and pulse, brought a shower seat, skin shields, and protective pad.

Tuesday, January 23

Mom slept until ten o'clock. She was very alert going into the shower, and she sat on the shower seat that Nancy brought. It was something different to her, so she was concerned about taking a shower with the seat there, but once Ginny coaxed her into the shower, she enjoyed sitting on it. Ginny said that it made it much easier to bathe her. She's still weak, and it would be easy for her to slip in the tub.

Dr. Kay called personally to let us know that the specialists who examined the results of Mom's hospital stay are in agreement that she probably doesn't have much more than two to four weeks to live, if that.

Wednesday, January 24

I sent e-mails to Gail and Fred, the Fitzgeralds, and the people closest to Mom whom I have been keeping informed of her situation on a regular basis since early October. I let them know that Mom is home with us for what will probably be, according to the doctors, the last few days—a month at most—of her life. I let everyone know that the cancer, which apparently began in a lung over a year or two ago, has spread to the liver, brain, and other parts of her body. We were blessed to have had her with us these past four months. I added that she is in no significant discomfort.

Gary called and said that he is coming up for a whirlwind twenty-four-hour visit this weekend. Everything is under control. Marli and Raina are so attentive to Grandma that it is a thrill just to watch them interact with her.

Raina knows Mom's entire daily routine (pills, cereals, prune juice, etc.) and doesn't hesitate to guide some of the more timid caregivers, although she is a bit more diplomatic, somewhat heeding our admonition to guide rather than order. Mom sits in our family room, takes everything in, chatters constantly, even though we don't understand much of what she says, and is so trusting in the way she follows instructions and reacts to attention that you just want to hug her and not let go.

We are all going thirty-six hours a day, instead of the usual thirty, to keep up on our work, to care for Mom, and to enjoy our little remaining time with her. Death is inevitable for all of us. Few of us are blessed, as we are, to have as wonderful an experience as our mother passes into the next life.

Obviously at some point soon we will have to deal with how to handle burial arrangements, whether to get an autopsy, hold the funeral in Florida, and so many other details. Gary and I discussed some of these issues, and he affirmed that he would speak with the people at Levitt-Weinstein Funeral Home and get back to me. He asked about the expanded options available for selection of caregivers now that hospice is involved.

I replied, "With the agencies, we have to take whatever caregivers they send. Most of the overnight people have been very good. Last night's caregiver, a new one, was okay but not on a par with others. Some of the weekend daytime people have been spotty. No one compares with Ginny, Betty, or Shirley; we really lucked out on Ginny when we needed someone the most—at the beginning. With agency people we can request the ones we like unless they're unavailable at the times we request them, in which case we have to take what we can get. So, yes," I concluded my response to Gary, "the expanded list from hospice, and their coverage of much of the cost, should significantly increase our chances of improving the quality of caregivers that we are limited to from the agencies."

Desiree is also very good with Mom, but sometimes she comes on a little strong, personally, in the way that she involves herself with the family. Maybe I am overreacting, because she has been really good. But one night while Susan and I were in bed watching TV, she came up the stairs and looked into our room to ask a question about Mom's care. I just felt that she could have yelled the question from the bottom of the stairs considering the hour. But I have no other complaints about her, and this one is minor—and who knows if maybe she did call up and we didn't hear her. The TV was on, and we may not have heard if she did yell to us before coming up the stairs.

Thursday, January 25

I keep checking forecasts in the hopes that we can encourage Gary to make the trip this weekend. He called to say that if it looks really bad, he can postpone for a week, but he'd hate to do that given how time is really marching on this situation. On the other hand, he has not driven in wintry conditions for years and is leery about getting in a situation where he is driving on slippery roads. I told him that the forecast sounded promising so far, and I would keep him informed and my fingers crossed. I suggested that I didn't mind picking him up and dropping him off at the airport. Even though the closest large airport is almost two hours away in Ottawa, Canada, it is an easy ride for me and one that I make fairly often.

Mom called everyone "Mary" today, including me at times. The rest of the family thinks this is hysterical since I'm usually the only one whose name she gets right. Yesterday Sue was Raina all day. Nonetheless, Mom did seem to know who we were, even when she couldn't match the right name with the person, and she obviously feels completely secure and trusting in this environment.

I received the following e-mail from Gail today:

"Good to hear from you but very sad news. You are lucky to have had some close times with your mom as indeed she is to have you. I have been very sad to hear about her deterioration as I, and indeed my whole family, have very fond memories of her. We all missed seeing her in Florida last month as we always have on our past visits, and it has been a very important part of our annual trips. Although we were grateful for the use of her apartment at Christmas, it felt very empty. I guess from what you have said, her rapid decline must be as much related to the cancer as to the Alzheimer's.

"We were shocked to see the state of my mother," Gail continued, "and indeed you were right about her deterioration. Unfortunately she is not as amenable or as accessible as your mom (no big surprise—she never was) and could hardly bear to think about it and certainly not with us. Mel got her to the doctor's, and she is on a drug called Aricept (if she is taking it). We had a fright when, on the first day, she took three tablets. It all feels very painful to me, not in the least because no one could talk about it. I thought Mel was very depressed, not surprisingly, but wouldn't let us talk about it with him and my mother together. I guess he was worried that she would think he was complaining about her. We would have liked to have talked to them about moving, but at the moment they were keeping private, and I guess we have to respect that. This getting old is really sad. Lots of Love, Gail"

I e-mailed Gail: "Yes, the mental deterioration through early November was probably due pretty much to the Alzheimer's, but the increasingly more rapid mental deterioration since then, and the physical deterioration, were due to the brain cancer. Now that she is on a pill to reduce swelling in the brain, her mental functions seem to be restored to the way she was in mid-November. She can respond to certain questions, and she can ask, 'Where are you going?' as you start to leave, and, 'When will you be back?' I don't think she can process the responses, but she knows to ask the right questions at the right times."

I concluded my e-mail to Gail, letting her know of a conversation I had with her mother. "I called your mother Tuesday afternoon, when we got the doctors' diagnosis, and I left a message on her answering machine that my mother had cancer, and the estimate was two to four weeks to live. She returned the call and spoke to Susan, who gave her more information and then put her on the phone with my mother. Nonetheless, last night your mother called again, and her opening comments were, 'Fred just called and gave me the tragic news about by my sister.' She apparently had no recollection of the two calls last week. Maybe, just as the Alzheimer's shielded my mother from the emotional trauma of coping with Ed's death, it may be helping your mom to escape what is happening."

At ten o'clock tonight, Mom started pointing toward me, and I couldn't figure out why. Finally I looked down and saw that my fly was open. I zipped it up, and she smiled and said, "Good."

Friday, January 26

It's incredible; Mom is actually getting stronger every day. I realize it is temporary and the result of the pills to reduce the swelling around the brain, but nevertheless, it is great. It means that she should be in condition to spend some quality time with Gary, who just confirmed that he will be flying into Ottawa tomorrow and will rent a car for the ride to Potsdam. For the past few weeks, Mom has looked so frail and has been able to walk only with assistance; sometimes it has taken two people to help her walk. Yesterday she was able to converse with us and understand some directions, as she would have a month ago. This morning, as I was grabbing some juice and talking with Desiree, the door opened to Mom's room. She was standing in the doorway, a big smile on her face. I said, "Good morning, Mom," and she said, "Good morning."

Fred called from Wyoming, and we talked for quite a while. He wanted to know if there was something he and Carole could do for his aunt Rhoda and our family. "Does your mom understand anything?" he asked. "If we were to send her something, would she enjoy it?"

"Yes," I replied, "she rereads the same cards over and over and over again. She appreciates flowers. Who can tell what she processes or retains, but she is aware when she is getting attention, whether it is through people, flowers, cards, or token gifts. That is why we keep her here. It is so obvious that she is aware of us, even when she mixes up our names."

I hung up the phone after talking with Fred, and I was walking into the family room when Ginny said to me, "Mom wants to know what you are selling."

"Mom, what do you want to buy?"

She smiled and said, in a hushed voice, "I don't know. What are you selling?"

"I'm selling to anyone, to anyone who will buy."

Mom pointed toward Sue, who was in the kitchen washing dishes. "Whatever she wants, I will buy!"

"Who is *she*?" I asked. Mom looked puzzled. "What's her name?" I persisted. Then Sue whirled around laughing, "Yeah, Mom, what's my name?" Mom laughed hysterically because we were all laughing, and she was part of it.

"That's Sue," Ginny said. "And I'm Ginny, even though you keep calling me Sue."

"That's right," Mom says.

It's worth it just to walk in the door and to see her look up, a smile broadening across her entire face, and hear her say, "Hi, Don!" One morning recently I walked into the room where she was seated with Ginny, and she said, "Hi!" I asked, "Who am I?" She responded, "You're Fosamax," the name of a pill she used to take each morning. But the recognition of me as someone who loves her was clearly evident.

Later in the day, Fred e-mailed again. His message was succinct: "It is so hard on families when everyone is so spread apart."

Sue was at book club, her oasis once a month from the hectic home/work/Mom/kids pace. This evening's fill-in caregiver, Kim, asked me, "Do you know where her pajamas are?" I looked in Mom's dresser drawers, couldn't find any, returned to the family room, and said, "I can't find them." Mom asked, "What are you looking for?"

"Your pajamas," I said.

"For you?" Mom asked.

"No, Mom, for you."

"Your pajamas for me," Mom said. "That's nice."

"No, Mom," I said. "Your pajamas for you. You'd look pretty silly in my pajamas."

Mom laughed. Kim continued walking Mom toward the kitchen, en route to her bedroom, and said, "Yea, hon, you'd look pretty silly in his pajamas, wouldn't you?"

"I guess so," said Mom, as they both laughed.

Saturday, January 27

Gary confirmed that he should arrive in Potsdam by late afternoon. This morning we were deluged with e-mails from close friends and relatives who received the update from me informing them of Mom's diagnosis and limited time to live. Carole e-mailed and said that Fred had filled her in. According to Carole her own parents are "visibly deteriorating, and my sister Deb and I visit frequently. They have around-the-clock aides. They turned down our offer four times to either move closer to Fred and me or to move near Deb in New York. Our visits are not really satisfying and are quite expensive." Carole concluded her e-mail by also offering, "If there is anything we can do, please let us know. We'll try and call you this evening. Love to Sue, Marli, Raina, and a special hug for Rhoda. You've been great children to your mom."

I sent an e-mail to Fred and expressed my appreciation for the thoughts expressed by him and by Carole. "Just the exchanges and knowing you are there is exceptionally meaningful. Every time I look at Mom, I conjure up almost sixty years of wonderful memories, starting with the ten of us at a table in Grandma and Grandpa's dining room and of so many other things that will keep us eternally close."

I received e-mails from my younger cousins, Diane and her younger brother, Lee Alexander. This is my father's side of the family through his sister, Vera. At the time I was born, The Alexanders' were living in Lawrence, Long Island not too many miles from Lynbrook. My mother and Vera had gone to the same summer camp as teenagers and became close friends. It was through Vera that Mom met my father. Before I was eight, the Alexanders' moved to Cleveland and then, three years later, to Akron, Ohio, where Vera's husband, Uncle Sam, opened what became a chain of "Home Center" stores. Uncle Sam retired in 1976 and he and Vera joined Lee in Tucson a year later where Lee had recently completed his last two years of college.

I was immersed in the importance of family from all sides. This was the highest priority of Susan's parents and, hence, the reason Susan felt so strongly about bringing Mom to Potsdam when Ed passed away. My grandmother Ruth, whose husband died in 1941, lived with Aunt Vera and Uncle Sam until her death in 1970 so Diane and Lee spent their entire childhood under the same roof with their maternal grandmother. Diane pursued a retail career in California until 2004 when she returned to Tucson to live with and care for her father after her mother died shortly before her 81st birthday.

Long after we were all grown, my cousin, Diane, told me (jokingly, I hope) how easy it would have been for her and Lee to have hated Gary and me. Since our father's parent, Grandma Ruth, was living with them in Akron, she only visited us in New York once or twice a year. However, when she came she would bring our all-time favorite spice cookies, a taste that seemed to have gingerbread and cinnamon flavor in an almost-cracker-like textured, diamond-shaped cookie. According to Diane, "Every time Lee or I would reach for a cookie out of the tin Grandma was filling, we'd feel a slap on the wrist and be told, 'Leave those alone; they are for Donnie and Gary.' It was enough to make us despise you both."

In her e-mail this morning, Diane wrote, "I don't know just what to say. I've been reading your updates, and they are beautiful and remind me of how we were with our mom. I think that the experience of being a family during this 'end-stage' is a gift. The memories of this time together will, I hope, be a comfort to everyone. I remember Aunt Rho as having a wonderful, dry sense of humor and intelligence. One of my fondest memories is of her voice. It was very musical and feminine. Mom loved to talk about your mom and dad. I think those days when they were all so young, so poor, and so in love must have been very happy ones. Marli and Raina are wonderful. They will cherish this time as they grow older. My thoughts are with all of you."

While I speculate whether my father or my paternal grandfather would have suffered from Alzheimer's if they had lived more than fifty-two years, there is no evidence of Alzheimer's on

Dad's side of the family. Both my father's mother, Ruth, and my aunt Vera died a few months short of their eighty-first birthdays, and they were both intellectually sharp right to the end. Grandma Ruth died from congestive heart failure, and Aunt Vera passed away in August of 1998 from heart and coronary artery disease (possibly the cumulative effects of years of smoking; she wasn't able to quit successfully until she was sixty-five).

Within minutes of hearing from Diane, this arrived on my computer from Lee: "How fortunate you are to be able to have her with you now. She is a wonderful woman. I have many fond memories of my childhood and being with her and your dad. Our hearts are with you. Please keep in touch! Lee & Family."

Mom was having a really good day, lots of dialogue. She called me Raina, and Raina loved it, but Mom is peppy, cheerful, and animated. She is eating better every day, too—some light solids. She seemed to understand when we told her that Gary was on his way, and I am hoping she stays on this plateau until Gary arrives and throughout his visit.

An e-mail arrived from Gail: "I just told Fred that we need to decide how and what and when to tell my mom about Aunt Rhoda's condition. Any thoughts?" I wrote back to Gail immediately, reminding her of the email I had sent her two days ago explaining that her mother already knew. "Gail, your mom has already been told several times. In my opinion, you can talk freely with her about it. She will not retain or process enough to cause harm, even though she will react dramatically each time you discuss it."

Carole wrote from Wyoming, and we proceeded to have an e-mail conversation:

"You guys are really terrific, and when Fred spoke with his mom last night, she expressed much gratitude for the way you're taking care of her sister. I think it is really hard for Millie to handle what has happened. From my experience with my mother-in-law, when things happen that she can't handle, she either denies them or forgets them. She's done that as long as I've known her—her way of coping I guess. This is why I think she acted like she had just heard about the cancer for the first time from Fred."

"Carole," I e-mailed back, "I understand exactly what you are saying. I recall a time when I was about twelve, and I was leaving for camp for two months, and I went next door to Aunt Millie's house to say good-bye. I walked in, and when she wasn't downstairs I began hollering, 'Is anyone home?' 'Come on up,' she yelled from her bedroom. When I got there and said I didn't want to leave without saying good-bye, she said 'Oh, I didn't come over because I hate good-byes; I'd rather just act as if you're not going away.' This always stayed with me because, at a young age, it struck me as a strange kind of self-deception for an adult to engage in; I was too young to realize adults have foibles just like children."

"For my own information," Carole asked, "how did your mom's doctor diagnose with such certainty that it is Alzheimer's? My dad's doctor said that the only way to do that is during an autopsy."

"We've been told that, technically, there is no diagnosis of Alzheimer's until an autopsy; however, an accumulation of symptoms can make a doctor almost certain. They call it dementia because of the fact that they can't ethically classify it as Alzheimer's until they do the autopsy. Carole, I can't be certain, but I think many of Aunt Millie's symptoms are exactly what my mom had a year ago. It is more difficult to tell with Millie because, as you say, she has always used memory loss as an escape from reality. However, when we ate with her and Mel every night for almost a week in late August, and again in late September, she had difficulty remembering things that had been said just moments before—and the kinds of things even absent-minded people don't forget. I've sensed the same thing on the phone with her in matters where there was no need to escape."

Carole wrote back, "My thoughts are constantly with all of you. I'm so happy that you are able to be together and involved near the end of your mom's life. You and your family have such generosity of spirit and conviction to follow through on what you know to be the right thing to do. I really admire all of you. Love to you all, Carole."

The support from Carole and so many others really does help keep us going and reinforces in me Susan's deeply held belief in the importance of family.

Gary arrived here for the start of his day-and-a-half round trip. Raina is thrilled to see her uncle Gary, as are we all. When he entered the house, Mom greeted him with a welcoming smile and a "Hi, Gary," giving evidence that she not only recognizes who he is but also that she knows he is someone special to her. Gary lowered himself toward the couch where she was seated, placed his hands on her hips, and kissed her on the cheek. Mom was visibly joyful. For the remainder of his brief stay, Gary engaged Mom in dialogue, and her responses were occasionally relevant to what he had just spoken and at other times didn't seem to be responsive, but they clearly indicated her pleasure that they were having a conversation.

I am grateful that he was able to squeeze in the visit because I know how difficult it would be for me to get away if Mom were in North Carolina and I had to juggle my business schedule with the difficulty of winter transportation to and from Northern New York. In some ways the lack of a major airport close to Potsdam makes it harder to travel between Potsdam and Chapel Hill than between major cities that are much farther apart. But it also means a great deal to me because a diminishing number of people share a lifelong connection with Mom, and this gives Gary and me a special bond at a time like this.

Mom had some of her better days Saturday and Sunday, and Gary enjoyed the visit.

Susan reminisces about her mother-in-law:
She would sit in our living room in the early evening with Ed and a group of our friends, and she would be enjoying the conversation, and at the same time she would be paying attention to Ed and snap her fingers at him. She explained that he picked his ears, and that snapping her fingers in his direction was a signal for him to stop.

Diane reminisces about her aunt:
Aunt Rhoda's musical voice still lingers in my mind! I can still see her smile as well.

Appreciating Mom Through the Lens of Alzheimer's

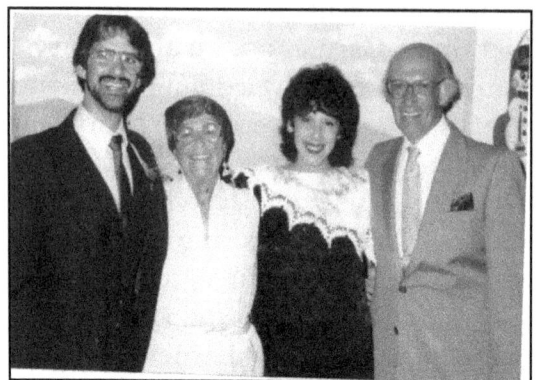

At left, Mom's sister-in-law (Harold's sister, Vera) with Uncle Sam, son Lee, and daughter Diane (approximately 1983).

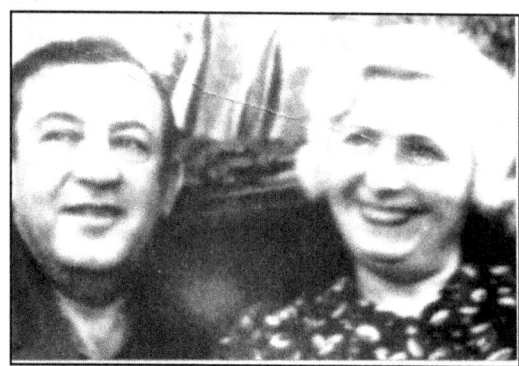

Don's paternal grandparents, David and Ruth Mesibov. David died of a heart attack at the age of fifty-two, two months before Don was born. Ruth lived with her daughter's family from 1941 until her passing in 1970.

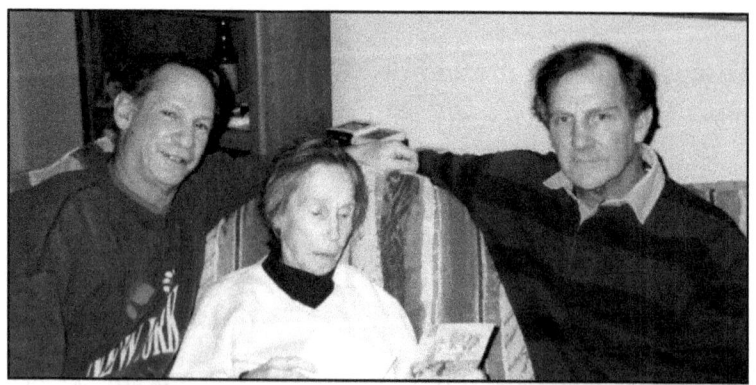

Sons Don and Gary flank Mom as the Alzheimer's and cancers take their toll.

A New Diagnosis: Four Weeks to Live

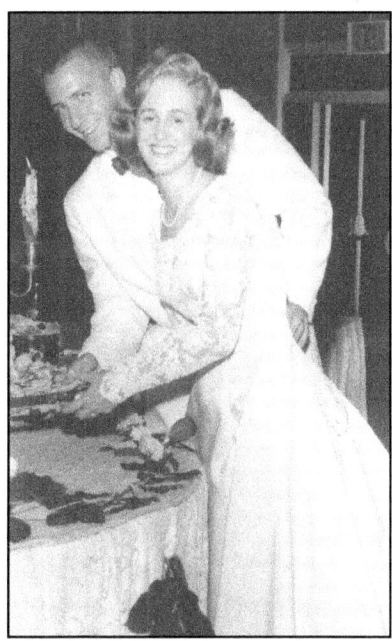

Cousin Fred and Carole on their wedding day June 10, 1962; they called and e-mailed frequently from their home in Laramie.

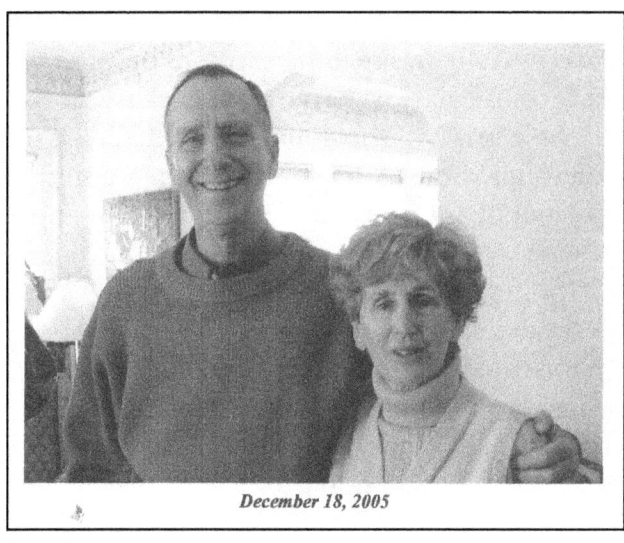

This is the last photo of Fred. It was taken shortly before he and Carole left Laramie for the Mayo Clinic in Minnesota December 19, 2005 where he died unexpectedly on January 1, 2006.

Chapter 14

The Patient Continues to Hold Her Own

Monday, January 29

Mom woke up early this morning and complained of a severe pain. Ginny, after calling Dr. Kay, gave her a dose of morphine.

Tuesday, January 30
Ginny's Journal:

When I arrived at 7:15 am, Rhoda was up watching TV with Desiree, and she was very alert, very talkative, and she was reading captions on the TV. She likes the musical kids' programs. For breakfast she had a whole bowl of wheatena—she fed herself some, and I fed her some. After breakfast she wanted to sit on the couch, and she watched TV for half an hour. Then she rested her eyes and talked to Darren.

Thursday, February 1

Mom was up until three in the morning, as talkative at night as she had been all day, according to Desiree. However, the long haul from seven o'clock Wednesday morning until three this morning, with only an occasional nap, exhausted her. She slept until 11:45 a.m. and got up for less than ninety minutes. At one this afternoon, she told Ginny, "I'm tired," and went back to sleep. She is still sleeping now at two thirty.

The Patient Continues to Hold Her Own

Monday, February 5
  Ginny's Journal:
    We did some walking and looking at photo albums. Rhoda recognized herself and Don and some other family members. Also pointed out Don once and said, "Donnie."

Tuesday, February 6

Late this morning Mom had about an hour of discomfort, and Ginny, again after calling Dr. Kay, gave her morphine. Mom was quite uncomfortable for about another hour, and Ginny gave her a second dose, and the pain apparently subsided. She has been fine all day since then. Later in the day, as I turned to walk away from Mom, she shouted after me, "Don, your futch is out." I turned, and she was pointing toward me. Sure enough, the tag on my sweatshirt was sticking out at the collar.

My usual correspondences to keep friends and family updated have been nil for the past week as I prepared for a major weekend conference (just held) and battled the flu simultaneously. Fortunately, Darren flew in for the week and has been an enormous help chauffeuring Marli and Raina to basketball, karate, concert choir, cello lessons, and piano lessons and even taking Marli and a friend of hers to Rochester yesterday for Marli to audition with a Saratoga group for a month-long summer program in New York City. Much of Darren's time this week, also, has been spent ridding our computers of the virus they've picked up; I guess the flu season isn't limited to people.

It has been a hectic week, but happily, despite the pain that was relieved with morphine, Mom has stayed on the plateau she reached when Gary was here. She is comfortable, chatty, smiles a lot, loves to read and reread cards, and is thrilled with the flowers she received from so many people. Her eating has picked up. Sometimes the caregivers are timid about encouraging her to eat. Then Raina takes over. "Grandma, you really do want to eat, don't you? Open your mouth, Grandma; that's it, open wide." Mom now seems to call everyone "Mary" most of the time but occasionally uses our correct names. I'm sure she knows who we are and from whom she is receiving things; she just can't connect the words with the thoughts she has much of the time.

The only contact we've had with the doctors since mid-January was when Mom felt a pain in her ribs and we spoke with the nurse. I guess I've been so surprised that she is still with us and doing so well that it hasn't occurred to me to speak with the doctors since we took Mom home from the hospital. They seemed so definite and so final in their prognosis.

Gary checked into some of the information I wanted him to find out from the funeral home. We can call Levitt-Weinstein or our local funeral home when the time comes. They will coordinate with each other. Levitt-Weinstein is a Jewish funeral home, and that, alone, will make it certain that any religious needs Mom would have wanted will be met.

We always leave the door to the cellar ajar so the cats can go downstairs to eat and to use their litter box. This drives Mom bats; the caregivers tell us she is constantly pointing as they walk by and insisting that the caregiver shut the door. Mom's sense of orderliness persists.

We had a rollicking dinner. Mom was cheerful, calling everyone Mary, as she does more and more—although she does alternate calling me Don and Mary. The kids can't let go of the Marys, and they think it is great that we all have the same name.

Thursday, February 8
Ginny's Journal:
Good mood; very alert. We did walking, played tic-tac-toe, and did some numbers. Raina was a big help. I printed my name, then Raina printed hers, and then Rhoda printed hers. We watched TV; she followed it closely, read everything, including a lot of numbers.

Friday, February 9

Gail e-mailed to say that she has been away and was worried about her aunt Rhoda due to the change in her diagnosis, and she asked to be called if her condition suddenly gets worse. She said that she would phone anyway to keep in touch, but "at times like this, we all seem so far apart."

Gary called to say that he would try to come up on the weekend of February 24, but he is having trouble switching coverage. He said that if Mom hangs in there, he will be up either that weekend or the one following.

Saturday, February 10

Leilani sent this sweet e-mail reminder of the many times she and Donald spent with my parents: "Had to laugh at your last update, especially the part that Rhoda is a stream of chatter, usually questions. Don, I think your mother was born chattering a stream of questions. I think she started asking questions of the nurses and doctors who delivered her. Her questions are what I remember most about her and loved so much in her. Over the years as I raised my two girls, I wished for her talent to ask questions. I don't think you and Gary were able to keep much secret from her when you were teenagers and young men. I suspect that in answering her, neither of you could totally keep track of her questions, and in the end, she knew a lot more than either of you thought you told her. Keep us posted on things up there. Love, L."

Sunday, February 11

Desiree's Journal:

Rhoda had been up all night. She said she had back pain. At 4:30 am I gave her morphine when she repeated how much it hurt. She got 0.25 ml of morphine.

Monday, February 12

On a positive note, this week has been much like the past few. Mom was alert, no deterioration of mental faculties, awake most of the time. She seemed to stay awake for long periods, with occasional catnaps, and then she slept for up to ten hours. Usually Mom's ten hours of sleep was at night. However, according to the caregiver, she was awake almost all Sunday night, went to sleep at six in the morning, and then slept until eleven. When I walked back into the house at one o'clock today, she was sitting up in the living room, looking through picture albums with Ginny. She had a nice, bright, "Hi, Don," for me, although most of the time we have all become Mary. "What do you think we should do with her?" she asked me, seriously, referring to Ginny. Knowing she doesn't usually understand the meaning of what she says, I replied, "Let's bury her." Mom laughed even before Ginny began laughing, so at times she does seem to understand a joke—or at least that a joke has been told. She was a constant stream of chatter when she was awake, usually with questions.

Tuesday, February 13

There were five or six times in the past week when Mom complained of pain, usually in the rib area, to the point where the caregiver administered a dose of morphine. It always happens either when we are out or in the middle of the night when we are asleep, so we haven't witnessed this yet. But she hasn't had any apparent pain yesterday or today. Her weight is down to eighty-five pounds, but she seems to eat well at every meal. Raina has become the master of convincing Mom to finish everything on her plate. "Come on, Grandma, you and I will both open wide and eat at the same time," Raina will say. "Okay," Mom will say, not moving. "You do it." "No," retorts Raina, "we both have to do it. Grandma, pick up your fork. Like this. Pick it up—that's right." We continue to have many laughs and good times. It is nice having her here and knowing that she is here.

Wednesday, February 14
Ginny's Journal:
Rhoda awoke at 8:30 am, and there was a strong urine smell. She was somewhat weak and disoriented going upstairs. Once in the bathroom the shower went very well and the hair wash. She really enjoyed the note that Raina left on the kitchen table for her before heading to school. "To Grandma for Valentine's Day." Also, we reread the Valentine cards from Gary and family and from Toby and from Gail. She enjoyed our game of tic-tac-toe today. When Susan, Marli, and Raina returned from school in midafternoon, they presented Rhoda with a large helium balloon on which is written, "I Love You."

Thursday, February 15
Betty's Journal:
Rhoda was at the dinner table when I arrived. I cooked potatoes with gravy and cheese, and she had pudding with medicine, and a small amount of yogurt. Very talkative. We did some walking and exercises this evening. Small piece of pie at 9:40 pm. Put Rhoda to bed at 10 pm. I got her up around midnight to go to the bathroom. She was lying across the two beds.

Friday, February 16
Ginny and Mom did some walking and looked at pictures. Mom identified family members such as Sue, the children, and me. Periodically, Mom kept reading and rereading aloud her "I Love You" balloon.

Sunday, February 18
We have had no instances of pain since Monday; the caregivers have not had to administer morphine at all. Mom slept eleven hours tonight.

Monday, February 19

Mom hardly slept at all tonight.

Tuesday, February 20

Frequent naps today. At one point, Ginny can't get Mom to sit up; Mom just doesn't seem to have the strength. However, Ginny and Sue eventually got Mom sitting up and then walking with some support. Ginny then took Mom for a walk as I held my breath, wondering if Mom had the strength to stand and walk. By dinnertime Mom was her usual cheerful self. She chattered away, loved being around people, and laughed often.

Wednesday, February 21

Gary called to let me know how much money we have left in Mom's checking account. He said that he was unable to arrange coverage for this weekend, but he will definitely come on the weekend of March 3. If I feel that Mom might not last that long, he will find a way to come this weekend, but I assured him that there has been little change in her condition over the past few weeks. I asked him if he has heard from his father-in-law, Dr. Levenson, about what we have to do about getting an autopsy. "Will notifying the funeral home take care of that, or is there another step for us to take?" He said that all we have to do is notify the funeral home, and they will take it from there.

Thursday, February 22

Darren has made two trips in the last three weeks to help us out. He spent four full days ridding both our computers of viruses, installing all kinds of protective software, and building us a firewall (whatever that is). He certainly doesn't get this talent from his father.

This past week Mom has called me Don about half the time, even Donnie a few times—the name she always used to call me but hasn't used much for the past few months. She also called Sue, Marli, and Raina by their correct names some of the time, called all of us Mary a lot, and has recently been calling us all Dorothy. Nonetheless, she clearly recognized everyone who was around her, felt completely secure, and was trusting as a child of us and everyone we brought into the home. She took delight even when the cats or Frisky curled up next to her, as they frequently did. Ginny said that her math ability has returned, and Mom can do addition, multiplication, and other functions that stump Ginny. She can't play games at the level of a few months ago, but Ginny has been able to get her back to at least playing some of these games.

Mealtime was our favorite time. At the start, the caregiver usually had to feed Mom, but by the end of the meal, with some coaxing and modeling by Raina, Mom was often feeding herself. Usually she'll have hot cereal, applesauce, or something soft.

She continues to lose weight, but now it is extremely gradual. She looks frail and may have difficulty surviving an illness of any kind, but we have been fortunate that she has remained healthy and seems to enjoy every minute that she is alive, as we enjoy her. I like the reinforcement when, forgetting Mom is even at the table, I may say to Raina, "You really need to focus more on your homework." Then I'll hear Mom assert, "That's right." Of course, there are also times when Raina may say, "I think I should be allowed to have another dessert," and Mom will also say, "That's right." These are the times Raina feels that Mom's word should be law. The past ten days have been good to all of us.

Friday, February 23

Sue met with the local funeral home director, and they discussed arrangements, when the time comes, for Mom's burial next to Ed in Florida. The airline requires a container; this will cost four hundred dollars. Sue called Gary, and then with his assent, she ordered one. Otherwise there would be a delay in getting it at the time it is needed. The container is a flying requirement, regardless of whether there is an autopsy or not. In addition to the four-hundred-dollar fee for the container, there is a three-hundred-dollar fee for the plane fare (these would exist without the autopsy); there will be a fee for the autopsy, and a fee for the funeral home. Most, not all, of these costs are covered by the policy Mom and Ed took out with Levitt-Weinstein. The two funeral homes—the one in Potsdam and Levitt-Weinstein—will handle everything once we call either of them. Ed set this all up years ago to protect us from bearing the cost of funeral and burial arrangements.

Saturday, February 24

Gary e-mailed that he will be in California this week, and he hopes to see cousin Diane during his visit. When I shared the news with the family that Uncle Gary will be here next weekend, Marli was thrilled, and Raina went through the roof with excitement. I e-mailed Gary: "While you have always been a favorite of hers, I think the time the two of you spent together in Florida last September solidified your MVP role in her life." He wrote back, "Tell Raina I am pretty excited about the trip as well."

Sunday, February 25

We had assumed that Mom's difficulties sleeping last fall were primarily due to the Alzheimer's. Often she stretches out across both beds, the trundle and one underneath that we brought up to the same level. Also, the caregivers have been sitting next to her just in case. Tonight, Mom was up on and off since midnight, and it is now six in the morning. Sue went downstairs to fill in for the caregiver whose shift ended at six, while she awaited the eight o'clock arrival of the next caregiver. Sue found Mom and the caregiver watching TV. The caregiver told Sue, "Rhoda won't go to sleep and keeps chattering away, so I finally decided it would be better to keep her occupied, and maybe she will nap for a long time during the day." The caregiver, her shift over, left. Sue turned off the TV and said, "Mom, would you like to go to sleep?" Mom smiled and said, "Sure." I think she would have said "sure" if Sue had asked if she wanted to go skiing.

Sue got Mom into the bed and lay next to her. Every couple of minutes, Mom said something, and Sue responded, "Shh, let's go to sleep." Finally, after half an hour, Mom went to sleep and stayed asleep for six hours. Sue's conclusion: Mom's restlessness in the autumn and early winter was sometimes due to not having anyone in bed alongside her. She was used to always having Ed in bed with her, and now, after twenty-nine years of marriage, she was alone in bed. This was having a disproportionate effect on her ability to fall asleep because of all the other disconcerting thoughts going on in her mind. We had noticed this inability to sleep when we were in Florida in September while Ed was in the hospital. Now when Mom has difficulty sleeping, the simple act of a caregiver, or Susan in this case, lying down in bed beside Mom seems to give her comfort.

Sue shared another observation, this one from Nancy Fletcher, the supervisor from hospice who visits and checks on Mom once a week. Nancy told Sue that it is not uncommon for Alzheimer's patients to survive cancer longer than others because others, knowing their condition, often give up on themselves sooner. Mom is clearly enjoying herself. She smiles a lot, chats constantly, asks us to come over when we are near, and enjoys our company and that of anyone who visits. And of course, she does not understand that she has cancer.

Gary called in the afternoon, and I shared Nancy's thought with him. "This is an especially interesting theory about why Alzheimer's patients might live longer with cancer," Gary observed.

Monday, February 26

Leilani e-mailed with an idea for helping Mom sleep. She said that she has heard that some medical professionals with patients who have lost a spouse provide them with a full-body pillow. They are longer than a king-size pillow—almost five feet in length. She said it might give Mom comfort. She suggested that we still may need the caregiver or Sue to shush her and quiet her down, but the pillow may help. It tends to give patients security, and further, they can put their arms around it and cuddle to it. I thanked Leilani for the idea and said that I would share it with Sue and the caregivers.

At bedtime, Raina asked me, "Why does Grandma have to die?" Obviously, I don't have a satisfactory answer, but as I watch Raina speak with Grandma continuously, play the piano for her, encourage her to sing along, and chide and prod her into eating food, it is clear to me that there is meaning and value in what is taking place for as long as it lasts. All of us will have memories that will last a lifetime, and our store of information and reflections will continue to grow.

Tuesday, February 27

Mom is sleeping nine to twelve hours nightly now. Today she was full of pep. I became even more acutely aware of how lucky we are when a graduate student called to ask for a copy of a book on teaching strategies that I use in class. When I dropped it off, the student said that she was taking a five- to six-hour trip to Brattleboro, Vermont, this weekend and wanted to read the book in the car. As we talked, she explained that she was going to her grandmother's funeral. Her grandmother had suffered with Alzheimer's for twelve years, "since I was about twelve years old," she told me. Then she continued, "I haven't seen her for twelve years because my dad wanted us to remember her as she had been. Once she lost her memory of who we were, about twelve years ago, she could get frustrated and also get verbally violent when she couldn't remember things. She wasn't pleasant to be around."

Mom is so cheerful in contrast to this graduate student's grandmother. "How old was your grandmother twelve years ago, when she suffered noticeable effects from Alzheimer's?" I asked her. "She was fifty-two. My grandfather is now seventy-four and is in excellent physical and mental condition."

I wonder if Marli's initial reluctance to have her grandmother live with us for fear she would not be the same person Marli wants to remember has changed since Mom has been with us. Marli is so wonderful with Grandma that it is hard to believe that she will not cherish and benefit from at least some of these memories as she grows older. To her credit, any reluctance she may still harbor about having her grandmother with us is not reflected in the slightest in the way she demonstrates her love with attentiveness and time.

I reminded Mom, "Gary is coming this weekend."

"Oh wonderful," she said, and she smiled. We've discussed Gary's pending visit several times, and she seems to understand, at some level.

The names of the week have been Darren, Mary, and Dorothy. Most of us were called one or more of these names much of the time, yet there were times when Mom called us correctly by our actual names. There was a knock at the door, and flowers arrived for Mom from Gail; Mom frequently looked at them, smiled, and commented. I e-mailed Mom's appreciation across the Atlantic.

Wednesday, February 28

Mom continued to hold her own—maybe a slight bit weaker, maybe slept a little longer relative to time awake, but basically the same. Despite a twelve-hour sleep last night, she really tested Ginny. She was lying on her bed as I walked in while Ginny was putting away clothes. "Look who's here," Ginny said. Mom answered, "I see," without even opening her eyes.

"Look," said Ginny.

"I am looking," answered Mom.

"No, you're not. You're not listening to me." Finally Mom opened her eyes and glanced back at me as she heard my voice. "Oh, Don, what's that behind your blah?" Sure enough, she had noticed the pen behind my ear.

"It's a pen, Mom."

"Where'd you get it?"

"Downstairs, in my office."

Mom seemed to notice everything and be highly alert to what was happening around her. Gary observed this when we were in the bank with her in Florida in September. It continued. While she was frequently not able to find the word to describe what she wanted to say, she heard everything that was said, usually had a response or a question, and was interested in everything around her. Tonight, as I tucked her in, I reminded her that Gary would be here this weekend. She immediately asked, "How's Laurie?" At times, she does not make these connections, but it is reinforcing to us when she does.

I kissed her and said, "I love you," and she said, "I love you too," with a bright smile. This is a ritual we have. I always say, "I love you," as I kiss her good night. She either says, "I love you too," or "Thank you," and always with a smile.

As we did the last time he planned a visit, Gary and I exchanged regular e-mails about the weather forecast and whether Gary wanted to rent a car at the airport or have me pick him up.

Thursday, March 1

Mom again slept through the night, and this morning she was awake, according to Ginny, by nine fifteen. To my relief, she was quite alert all day. I was afraid the twelve hours of sleep the night before, followed by frequent naps and then another long night of sleep, might be a sign of regression. She seems to be settled into a nice pattern of lengthy sleeps at night followed by days that are mostly full of pep and being alert.

I e-mailed the latest weather report for the next four days to Gary. The temperature range was forecast to be from six to twenty-seven degrees, with the possibility of snow flurries over the weekend.

I let him know that there don't appear to be any major storms on the horizon. Gary replied, "Unfortunately, it turns out to be a work weekend, so I will have to stay at the nearby hotel where there is an Internet connection, and I can set up the computer and contact my person working with me in North Carolina when I arrive. Arrival at your home should be around four o'clock."

Mom was upbeat today and kept saying to Marli, "I love you." Marli responded each time, "Good, Grandma, I love you too." Grandma repeated, "I love you," and Marli kept repeating, "Good, Grandma, I love you too." This continued at least five minutes until Marli noticed the balloon hanging from the ceiling—which Sue had brought home for Mom on Valentine's Day—that says, "I love you."

Mom still loves to read. Frequently, she will blurt out "Watertown Daily Times," or "Bush Proposes Tax Cut," or something else that will indicate that she is reading something on the table or wall in front of her. Now she often blurts out, "I love you," as she gazes at the balloon, which either she hadn't noticed since mid-February, until today, or maybe it had only recently floated into view from a less visible part of the room.

Marli reminisces about her grandmother:
The quality I admired most in her was her patience. She'd sit with me for hours, letting me introduce her to all my stuffed animals.

Brian reminisces about his grandmother:
She always had a positive and upbeat attitude whenever we spent time with her. Even when we just talked to her on the phone, the Florida sunshine came through in her voice.

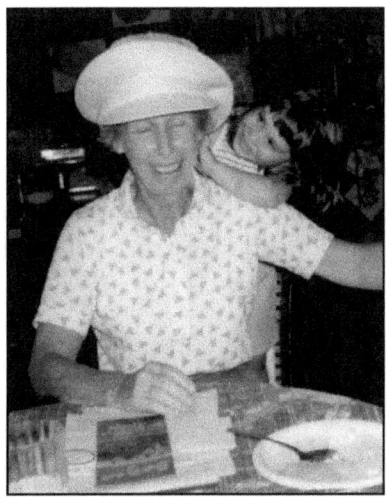

Mom's delight, and patience, with her grandchildren was always evident as in this picture with Marli.

Chapter 15

Simone, the Incompetent Caregiver

Friday, March 2

We continue to be sustained with supportive e-mails and phone calls. Fred wrote: "Thanks for letting us know how things are going. Carole has been dealing with arrangements for her parents. There are no good solutions when they are at such an advanced age. I pick up Carole at the airport today, and this coming Thursday we go to a cities conference for a few days and then head down to Florida to see my mother and Mel. That takes us to the end of our spring break. My book, *Primo Levi and the Politics of Survival*, is projected to come out in July."

Leilani sent another warm e-mail: "Thank you again for sending your updates. We so enjoy reading them. What is happening in your home is a most rare experience in today's world—love in bloom. How lucky all of you are to share in it."

Most of our caregivers are terrific, certainly the ones we use on a regular basis, but we have had some lemons. Ginny asked for today and Monday off because her daughter and son-in-law are visiting from out of town. But she made it clear that if we were unable to get someone through an agency, she would come. Desiree agreed to stay until noon to cover for Ginny, and Med Link promised it would provide a new person, Simone, from noon until four o'clock today, at which time Betty would arrive. Betty would stay on until ten tonight, and then Shirley was scheduled to come in until six in the morning, when Betty will return for an all-day Saturday shift.

At noon Simone arrived, and it soon became apparent that she doesn't enjoy this type of work. When Marli and Sue returned home from school at 3:40 p.m., Simone put her coat on and headed for the door. Sue reminded her that she was scheduled until four, and Sue needed these twenty minutes to get settled after a full day of work. A moment later, after Mom had addressed three comments in a row toward Simone—without any acknowledgement, much less a response—Marli turned to Simone and said, "Grandma is talking to you; don't you hear her?"

Simone responded, "I've been talking to her all day; why don't you talk to her?" I resolved to draft a letter of complaint to Med Link outlining the causes of our request that Simone not be sent again.

Tonight at eleven thirty, I returned from picking up Marli at a friend's house. Shirley was in Mom's downstairs bedroom putting her to sleep, so I missed my chance to pay her for the week. I figured I would have to catch up with her the next time she came, although that may not be for a few days or even a week.

Saturday, March 3

It was shortly before six when I was awakened by a few quick, loud barks from Frisky, which meant that Betty—arriving to take over from Shirley—was coming up the long driveway. While Frisky had gotten me up earlier than I wanted, it did give me a chance to catch Shirley before she left, so I grabbed my bathrobe and raced downstairs, cash in hand. As I entered the kitchen, Shirley and Mom were seated at the kitchen table, talking, and Betty was at the other end of the family room, taking off her coat and boots and getting settled.

"Your mother is a magnificent person!" Shirley announced.

"What kind of night did she have?" I asked.

"She slept from ten thirty last night until a little while ago. Occasionally I would hear her through the intercom, talking, and I would respond. She might say, 'What are you doing?' and I would say, 'Not much,' or she might say, 'Let's have a factory,' and I would say something to let her know I was here. But for the most part, she slept through, and she didn't get up at all."

"That's right," Mom said smiling, ever alert to any discussion taking place within earshot.

"Before she went to bed, and since she's been up, she has been reading a lot," Shirley told me. "She reads posters on the wall, newspaper headlines, and anything she sees. She's always asking me questions and commenting about everything. She's so cheerful. Your mother is a magnificent person."

Betty, who came in after Simone at four o'clock yesterday and returned this morning, is absolutely wonderful. She has the patience of the proverbial saint, always smiling, always pleasant. She brings her crocheting and has sparked an interest in Raina, who has taken up crocheting because of Betty's influence, and she is now making a blanket for her nana, Ruth. Raina works continuously on the blanket (we have to pull her away to do homework) and frequently says, "Won't Betty be surprised when she sees how much I have done?"

This morning Betty gave Mom a sponge bath, explaining, "I didn't want to take her upstairs to bathe because I didn't want to wake you, Susan, or the children."

Betty is soft-spoken and could convey the impression that she has been a "local" all her life, but she is far better traveled than I, having been a missionary overseas, among her exploits. She is missing the tip of an index finger, which Raina explained to us: "She sliced it off three days before her fiftieth birthday." Raina was obviously intrigued by this event and had been given a very patient and worthwhile education by Betty.

I came downstairs at about nine, having returned to bed for some sleep after paying Shirley, and Mom and Betty were at the breakfast table. Mom had a glass of juice in front of her and immediately looked up and said, "Hi, Don."

"She always lights up when you come into the room," Betty said to me. "In fact, when any members of the family come into the room."

"That's right," Mom said.

"Do you like having us around, Mom?" I asked playfully.

"Oh, sure." She smiled and then asked, "What's that factory?"

"It's just something I carry around," I replied.

"Oh good," Mom responded. Then she looked at Betty and said, "Isn't that nice, Betty? He carries it around."

Betty smiled broadly. "Did you hear that?" she asked me.

"Yes," I replied. "She called you Betty. Does that surprise you since that's your name? Do most people call you Dorothy, or Mary, or Gary?" I continued, teasing Betty. Betty laughed. Mom, seeing us laugh and banter, smiled and then began laughing too.

"Betty's amazed that you called her Betty," I said to Mom.

"Oh really," answered Mom. "That's nice."

Raina walked into the room. "Drink your juice, Grandma," she chided.

"I will," said Grandma, but she did not move a muscle to follow through.

"Drink it now," Raina repeated. "Like this." Raina picked up the cup and simulated drinking.

"That's nice." Grandma said, smiling.

"Now you do it, Grandma." Raina then picked up Grandma's hand, put it around the cup of juice, and started lifting it toward Grandma's mouth. As the hand moved a few inches off the table, Grandma took control, and Raina was able to let go as Grandma finished taking the cup to her lips and drank.

"Mom," I asked, "do you remember who's coming today?"

"No, who's coming?"

"Guess," I said, knowing that in the book *The 36-Hour Day* it warns not to do this because it can confuse and lead to frustration but also knowing that Mom will take this as a game and enjoy the banter.

"Which of your sons do you think is coming?"

"Yes," Mom answered, "which?"

"Is it Bob, Gary, Bill, Mary, or Sid?" I pressed on.

"That's a lot of sons," Mom responded.

"Gary is coming," I told her. "Won't it be nice to have us all together?"

"Yes, the whole family—it will be nice."

Sue entered the kitchen. Mom noticed her, turned toward her, and said, "Who's that, Raina?"

"That's me, Mom," Sue responded, used to being called a variety of names, but as we all do, responding whenever it is clear that Mom is talking to her.

"How are you this morning?" Sue asked.

"I'm fine, how are you?"

Yes, as Shirley said, Mom is a magnificent person. Shirley, other caregivers, and other guests to the house appear to pick up on Mom's wonderful personality and genuine love of life and people, despite the fact that she is unable to process information or fully comprehend what is being said. There is obviously an essence of Mom that comes through, despite being only eighty-one pounds and having an inability to…I was about to say communicate effectively, but I realize that she does communicate extremely effectively. What I guess I mean is her inability to communicate with the words and expressions to which most of us are accustomed.

Gary arrived around four o'clock. While smiling as she greeted him, Mom asked, "How's Laurie?" Gary stayed through dinner and until ten that evening, headed for a nearby motel that had the Internet connections for the work he needed to do while on the road, and returned early the next morning.

Sunday, March 4

Gary stayed to see the first half of Raina's middle school basketball league game before heading for the airport and concluding his whirlwind twenty-four-hour visit. Before he departed he offered to return the first weekend in April to cover for us when we will be heading to Briarcliff Manor for Seders to celebrate the first two nights of Passover.

The visit with Gary was nice for all of us. Mom clearly recognized him and enjoyed seeing and speaking with him. We all had fun together.

Monday, March 5
    Desiree's Journal:
        Rhoda was very sloppy last night. She was unsteady on her feet. I had her to bed at 9:30 last night, and she slept through."

Mom's sleeping habits have changed significantly since she first came to Potsdam, when she could barely stay in her room for more than half an hour at a time between ten at night and three in the morning.

Raina sent an e-mail to her uncle Gary just before she left for school with the subject, "*Guess what my whole basketball team got—GOLD MEDALS!*" Her message read, "Dear Uncle Gary, look at the picture I've attached. Isn't it exciting? It shows a hoop with a basketball going in. How was your trip home? Have fun! Raina."

A predicted snowstorm was starting as Betty—affable and competent, as usual—came in to replace Ginny, who was spending the day entertaining out-of-town family. Betty started up the stairs with Mom but couldn't get her past a few steps, came back down, and gave her a sponge bath instead of the bath she wanted to give upstairs in the tub. Also, as they walked into the living room later in the day, Mom became a little short of breath, quicker than usual—perhaps another sign of minor deterioration. Shortly after lunch, Shirley called to say that she couldn't make it in for the night shift because of the snow. She has a child with muscular dystrophy for whom she has to be home by 6:30 a.m., so she can't risk the possibility that the roads may become impassable later on; we had speculated that she might not make it in. Betty agreed to stay all night, which gave her a shift of more than twenty-four hours.

When Gary got Raina's e-mail this morning, he replied almost immediately. It was good that he did because Raina asked as soon as she got home from school if there was an e-mail response from Uncle Gary. "My trip home was fine, though I wish I could have seen the rest of your game. The first half was very fun, and you did very well. The picture of the hoop with the ball going through IS very exciting!!!"

Mom napped briefly in the afternoon and then joined us at the dinner table; everyone's mood was jocular. With snow now predicted to continue through the entire night, Betty and Raina have been crocheting away. But at dinner, we all stopped what we were doing while five of us had pasta, and Mom ate her pudding, having eaten her main meal for lunch.

We ribbed each other a lot, and Mom was quick to jump in, at appropriate times, with "That's right," or "She did," or "I didn't know that."

Tuesday, March 6

Mom woke up after a thirteen-hour sleep. She was alert, dialogued a lot (sometimes it was nonstop), and occasionally she called us by our correct names. Other times she said, "Raina, Raina, Raina," when Raina was nowhere around. One time Mom was looking straight at Susan. "Raina Susan." I yelled, "she's calling you. You're the Raina she wants right now." "What is it, Mom?" Susan asked. "That's nice," Mom responded.

Wednesday, March 7

I sent the following letter of complaint to the case manager at Med Link:

Fax to: Regina M. Randall, RN Case Manager
From: Don Mesibov
Date: March 7, 2001

Dear Ms. Randall,

We appreciate that you were able to provide coverage on Friday, March 2, and we realize we did not afford you much lead time; however, I want to report that Simone was completely unsatisfactory:
1. She arrived half an hour late.
2. A colleague called me that evening, and his exact words were, "You may want to rethink who you are using as a

caregiver." He had telephoned and tried to leave a message for me. Simone had obviously conveyed an attitude to him that caused a complete stranger to comment on her performance based on how she responded to him on the phone.
3. When my wife arrived home at 3:40 p.m., Simone began putting on her coat and preparing to leave. Was she not aware she was expected to provide coverage until 4:00 p.m.?
4. The previous caregiver had made lunch for my mother and had left sauce and noodles on the stove so that all Simone had to do was serve the lunch and feed my mother. Simone did feed my mother, but she left the sauce on the stove, did little clean up, and allowed the leftover sauce—a considerable amount—to spoil.
5. The attitude toward the job, conveyed by Simone to my wife, was one of little enthusiasm. She seemed to have an "attitude" problem.

Since October we have experienced at least six extremely competent caregivers, several of them hired through Med Link. Each of them has indicated my mother is a delight to care for and is less trouble than any patients they have handled. We appreciate the invaluable service provided us by Med Link; I thought you would want to know of this instance where performance was less than satisfactory.

Sincerely,

Don Mesibov

Thursday, March 8

Ginny told us that Mom seemed to be in pain when urinating—also with her BM. We called Nancy at hospice; she suggested that we encourage Mom to drink a lot of water. Mom walked more today, wandering around the main floor, reading whatever she spotted on the walls, tables, bulletin board above Sue's desk, or the refrigerator. She was able to feed herself the entire day.

Friday, March 9

Regina, the supervisor for Med Link, was here to give Mom an evaluation. We brought down the upstairs bathroom scale, and Betty and Regina helped Mom onto it. I took one look at the scale and yelled, "Mom, CONGRATULATIONS, you weigh eighty-five pounds!" We all cheered. Mom laughed and said, "Thank you."

"Mom," I exclaimed, "we are all celebrating. Raina deserves credit for taunting you and modeling so that you will eat. Betty deserves credit for not listening when you say, 'I'm not going to eat that.' You deserve credit for eating and taking all this guff from us." Mom smiled and said, "Ha!" We all applauded and cheered again. "Mom," I said, "If you get back up to a hundred pounds, we are going to put you on a diet."

"Oh, really," she said.

"Well, you're doing really nice," I said.

"I am?" responded Mom. "Thank you."

"Did you hear that?" Mom said to Betty. "I'm doing it." Betty laughed, perhaps thinking of the hour or more she often spends at the kitchen table with Mom, coaxing her to eat everything on her plate, sometimes getting Mom to feed herself, and occasionally having to feed her.

When Mom is awake and at the table or on the couch with us, there appears to be no slippage from a month ago. And since she left the hospital about seven weeks ago and began taking the pill that reduces swelling in the brain, I think she has maintained a pretty even keel. The rise in weight from eighty-one to eighty-five pounds is the first time she has gained weight since she began losing precipitously in December from a high of one hundred. We didn't think she'd ever gain any of it back. But I can see the slippage when I think that in October she was dialoguing mostly in cohesive sentences that said something, even when she would often repeat a request for information that had just been given. Until December, Sue or I would take her with us on trips to the store or to the mall, where we would take walks. Mom has not been out of the house since we returned from the hospital in January. If the weather warms, she could go out on our back deck, but trips to town, to the store, or anywhere out of the driveway are pointless. They would require too much effort from Mom and would not be enjoyable for Mom or us.

In December, Mom was still walking of her own volition and almost as well as when she and Ed used to take their daily walks. Now it takes up to two people to help her up the stairs for a bath. It is an effort for her to get up from the couch, with help, or into or out of bed. But her vocal tone, while softer, and her reaction to stimuli remain strong. "Who's that?" she'll immediately ask the caregiver if she hears the door to the house open. If I say, "I'll see you later, Mom," she seems to understand because she will wave good-bye or at least stop talking and expecting a response. "Where are you going?" she may ask when she sees me with my coat on.

Saturday, March 10

This morning I started to lose my footing in the family room, and Mom immediately said, "Whoops, watch out." Whether this represents understanding or it was simply a reflexive response, who knows? It continues to baffle us, trying to determine what she can and cannot understand. Clearly, if you were to say to Mom, "You have cancer," she would not begin to comprehend that there was anything wrong. She would react as if you had said, "You have a candy bar." She would either say, "Oh, is that right?" or "That's nice," or "Really?" So why does she know to say "Whoops" when it is the appropriate reaction?

When Mom first came here on October 4, she had to take more than fourteen pills a day between her memory pill, vitamins, calcium, etc. Just before the MRI that resulted in the cancer diagnosis in the hospital in January, the doctor eliminated all pills and then added just the pill to reduce the swelling of the brain, to be taken twice a day. I guess the doctor believed his two- to four-week prognosis for Mom's survival because he gave us a short supply of pills and marked "No refills" on the container. Monday we will have to call the doctor and ask for a new prescription. Happily, Mom has outlasted all predictions.

Monday, March 12
   Shirley's Journal:
   7 am - Rhoda sleeping on my arrival. Up at 8:50, a bed bath—alert—talkative; Rhoda seems quite weak while walking to kitchen this am—breakfast: banana, bowl of oatmeal, ½ yogurt, ½ dex (meds), ½ prune juice, water. Right elbow quite bruised, left elbow bruised also! It might be from eating, leaning on right elbow a lot lately.

Wednesday, March 14
   Ginny's Journal:
   Rhoda seems extra tired and a little confused while eating. Very good mood—talkative, walked—looked at picture album, walked, sat in rocking chair—feet are swollen at 12:30; feet hadn't been swollen this morning; elevated feet on pillows (removed shoes for a while). Lunch: homemade chicken noodle soup, ½ cup milk, pudding, water, 1 glass. Walking, tic-tac-toe. Looking at cards Rhoda received from Gary and the Fitzgeralds. Down at 5 pm.

Thursday, March 15
Nancy from hospice arrived for her weekly evaluation of Mom. She asked if we needed anything, and I said, "Why don't you bring a wheelchair just so we will have it." She indicated that she would also bring an oxygen tank, just in case. Sue immediately said, "Maybe we shouldn't get the wheelchair yet. If the caregivers see it, they may be tempted to put Mom in it rather than exercise her." "We'll hide it upstairs," I said, "so that when we do need it, it's here, and we don't have to wait a few days for it."

Friday, March 16
Mom was very alert, and according to Ginny, she seemed stronger today. She sat on the couch in the family room and walked with assistance.

I received this e-mail from cousin Diane: "When I read your letters, I feel like I am in the room with you. I can hear your mom's responses so clearly! Hugs to Raina; this can't be easy for her, but what an incredible experience to have. I am sure that both Raina and Marli have made a huge difference in how well Aunt Rho is doing. You and Susan are wonderful."

Physically, Mom has suffered serious deterioration, which leads me to question how much longer she can continue. On the other hand, her disposition and mental approach are about the same. In other words, when you sit and converse with her, she is back to the higher levels she had reached after her release from the hospital in January, once the pill for the brain cancer had been prescribed and had taken effect. Also, she continues to be able to eat well, not to gag, and is able to swallow, so maybe the physical deterioration is limited to those things that affect her mobility.

Gary recently commented that it is mysterious how the disease selects the functions that it does.

Saturday, March 17

Susan and I took Marli and Raina to Ottawa for an overnight. We were a little bit nervous about Sunday because that was the only day when the agency provided coverage, and that is usually when we get the weakest caregivers. The rest of the week, except for a few hours on Wednesday evenings, are covered by private caregivers whom we have hired, including some from the list provided by hospice. Ginny, Betty, Shirley, and Desiree are all terrific, as are a few others. They exercise Mom, talk with her constantly, cajole her into eating and into feeding herself, and really enjoy being with her. All four have established warm relationships with our children. Desiree, who was on duty last night, had flowers delivered for Marli two weeks ago with a note wishing her well in her weekend performances as a singer in a musical revue put on by students in her high school.

The four of us left for Ottawa in the afternoon to see Dionne Warwick perform that evening. Then we went backstage to meet her. Sue's uncle Stanley, who died two days after Marli was born, had made his living flying small planes, and he used to fly the singer around the Northeast for some of her concert appearances. As we waited for Ms. Warwick to come out of the dressing room, some of the orchestra members passed. Marli struck up a conversation with the cello player, and pretty soon, the cello player was taking the case off her cello and showing her instrument to an admiring Marli. Sue then spotted the trumpet player (a very talented young lady who had been featured at a previous concert we had attended in Ottawa), and then Raina was being asked questions by the trumpet player. When Ms. Warwick appeared, we had a nice conversation; she remembered Uncle Stanley and spoke fondly of her travels with him. We had our picture taken with her, and she asked that we send her a copy.

Sunday, March 18

We stayed in a hotel and called home at seven thirty this morning, just before Desiree was to go off duty. Everything was fine, according to Desiree. We called again at two thirty, when Nicole was on duty. Nicole is new, had been with Mom the previous Sunday for the first time, and is probably the one a CareGivers representative told us had called to complain that Raina was telling her what to do. We had decided to try this new agency after dissatisfaction with some of the caregivers sent to us by Med Link.

Susan asked about five questions; among them, has Mom eaten well, is she comfortable, and has she napped? Nicole assured Susan that everything was fine.

We called again at four thirty, and Mildred was now on duty, having taken over from Nicole at three. Mildred said that Nicole indicated that she had lots of problems with Mom. Also, Mildred told Sue that Mom was in the wheelchair when she arrived, and she said that she has a bad back and therefore can't care for someone who needs to be lifted in and out of a wheelchair. She informed Sue that she had called CareGivers, and they were sending a replacement for her. Also, CareGivers wanted me to call their office when I got home.

"Why is she in the wheelchair?" Sue asked Mildred. We didn't even realize that the wheelchair had been delivered by hospice. We later learned that Nancy had dropped off the wheelchair on Friday, while Ginny was on duty, and Ginny had put it in a corner of our dining room, a room that neither Mom nor caregivers need to be in. Mildred told Sue that all she knew was that Mom was in the wheelchair when she arrived at three on Sunday, and Nicole complained about having had lots of problems with Mom. I was frustrated and angry, and as soon as we got home early Sunday evening, I called CareGivers.

The lady on duty who answered the phone started out on the offensive and wanted to know why we hadn't told them that Mom was now wheelchair bound. Pretty soon I had her on the defensive. "She does not need a wheelchair," I stated, emphatically, and a lot louder than was necessary for her to hear me. "She never should have been put in the wheelchair. We had the wheelchair brought in just so it would be here when we eventually will need it." I also stressed that I was upset that Nicole had assured us that everything was all right, when apparently she felt it wasn't.

By now the CareGivers representative was apologizing, and I told her, "Most of our caregivers call us if they even have a question about which soup to feed Mom. In this case we called Nicole, and she assured us that everything was okay. She never mentioned any problems; she never said that she wanted to put Mom in the wheelchair." The lady from CareGivers explained that Nicole was new, and she apologized and promised that they will speak with Nicole. I repeated that we had left cell phone and hotel room numbers, and that either Nicole or Mildred could have reached us at any time.

Once again she apologized. And she said she felt badly for Mildred, who had traveled half an hour to our house only to have to leave ninety minutes later because she thought Mom was wheelchair bound. I couldn't resist a dig, and so I said, "You know, I'm not justifying that our ten-year-old was telling Nicole what to do a week ago—and we've told her not to do that—but the fact is that sometimes Raina is better able to understand Mom's needs than some of the caregivers we are sent. I can't understand why Nicole didn't pick up the phone and call us if she felt that Mom was having problems or needed a wheelchair. At the very least, she should have been candid when my wife asked her how Mom was doing."

When I got off the phone, we took the wheelchair upstairs and put it in the room Mom initially occupied, a room we keep closed during the winter to avoid wasting heat. We probably will need the wheel chair in a week or two. Mom needs a lot of help getting up out of a chair or back down into it; this has only been occurring recently. Ginny said that Mom has to be told to swallow at times because she will hold the food in her mouth and not try to swallow.

Darren flies in tomorrow, for a week. We welcome his ability to chauffeur the girls and to occupy them and Mom for as long as he is willing and able to apply his considerable expertise. His visits have provided valuable and welcome relief for us all. His sisters adore him and love having him around. They turn their schedules topsy-turvy to be with him, and they all have lots of fun together. And of course, we love having him with us, even when there is no reason for a visit other than to be with us.

Monday, March 19

Darren arrived, and Mom clearly recognized him, even though she couldn't recall his name. She lights up whenever she sees him, and he is very definitely warmed by her reception. It would be nice if everything could continue as it is, even with Mom's condition remaining the same. We know it can't; it could end any day. But each extra day is one more than we had been told to expect. Darren checked out all our technology. I can now relax, knowing that if one computer breaks down, I won't lose all my records and business files. The family is used to my panic attacks (and rotten moods) when the computer freezes and I fear that everything I am working on will be lost, my business will go down the drain, and I'll be forced into retirement.

Thursday, March 22

Mom's feet were still swollen. Nancy from hospice visited in the morning and informed us that the swelling seemed to be spreading slightly up the legs. So Nancy called the doctor, and he gave us a new prescription to replace the diuretic. Nancy said that the brain cancer could be causing the swelling in the feet, and it also could be making it more difficult for Mom's brain to send the commands to her feet when she is asked to stand or walk. It's hard to know how this is affecting Mom. In other words, is Mom reluctant to walk because of discomfort in the feet, or is the hesitant walking due to the brain not sending commands to the feet as quickly as usual?

Betty has noticed that sometimes it takes longer to get Mom to pick up her silverware and to use it because of a slowness in the brain in terms of issuing commands to hands. The good news is that, except for whatever discomfort the swelling in her feet is causing, she doesn't appear to be in pain. The forgetting to swallow is infrequent and not yet a problem, and while the exercise and walking are extremely limited from what they have been, Mom still can move around, usually needing help. She still eats well and continues to smile. Mom has only experienced serious pain a few times in the past two months. By the evening, Betty said she thought that the swelling in the feet was down a little.

Saturday, March 24

Betty got behind Mom, put her arms under Mom's shoulders, and tried to lift her out of bed this morning. This is the only way the caregivers can sometimes, safely, lift Mom. Betty pulled a little too hard, and Mom said loudly (loudly for her, but what would be considered softly for anyone else), "Ouch, that hurts." So we know Mom will tell us if there is pain, and that's why we're positive that, with this one exception, we've seen no signs of discomfort recently.

I came up from my basement office and into the kitchen at about ten this morning, and Mom was sitting at the table with Betty. "Hi, Mom," I said, "How are you?"

"I'm fine," she said, breaking into a broad grin.

"You're looking good, Mom. Are you taking good care of Betty?"

"Sure," Mom replied, still smiling. "I am."

In the supermarket this afternoon, I saw Mildred, the caregiver with the bad back. She asked about Mom. She also told me that when she had arrived at our house last Sunday, Mom had immediately greeted her with, "Hi, Millie." The past two weeks everyone has been either Marli or Raina to Mom—except that I was often called Don. For her to call anyone Millie—much less someone whose name is Millie—was unusual. Did Mom know this was Millie? Did she remember Mildred because it is her sister's name?

Coincidentally, when I got back from the supermarket, Aunt Millie called and expressed frustration that there is so little she can do to help her sister. She asked if Mom would recognize her if she came for a visit. I told her that I thought she would, although she may or may not call Millie by name. Aunt Millie decided the climate would be too cold for her. I suggested maybe in a month. At first she liked this idea, but then she decided that the airport is too far from our home. I suggested that we could pick her up, and, at first, she liked this idea, but then she decided it would inconvenience us, and, besides, "There will be no place for me to stay."

Sue overheard our conversation, took the phone, and offered our house or a very nice motel three miles away, and the decision on that was put off with, "Let me think about it." But Aunt Millie did ask about sending flowers.

Sunday, March 25

Today Darren fixed the sink, built some shelves, and designed some furniture he'll build for us next visit. Tomorrow, he and I will drive three and a half hours to Albany for his flight back. Marli came downstairs at ten o'clock, late for Sunday school where she teaches. When I asked her if it was her I heard coming up the stairs at 4:45 a.m., she thought for a minute, realized she couldn't—or shouldn't—deny it, but explained that it was Darren's last night here (well, tonight is, but she has school tomorrow), and that she wanted to spend the time talking with him and working together on the computer.

Monday, March 26
   Ginny's Journal:
      Rhoda was sleeping when I arrived. Sleeping later again today. Up at 11:20 am—bed bath—applied lotion all over, and A+D ointment on red spots on ankles, and bottom looks a little red. Rhoda's eyes look very red and look very sore. She's wearing her sunglasses. She is very tired and shaky. I talked to Nancy on the phone. Mary O'Brien, another RN with hospice, will be coming tomorrow with support hose, chuks, and gloves. Mary will also be here next week since Nancy will be out of town for the next two weeks.

Tuesday, March 27
   Mom's eyes were worrisomely red, and the swelling in the ankles and feet continued, so Ginny called Doctor Kay and set up an appointment for tomorrow.

Wednesday, March 28
   Ginny and I took Mom outside the house for the first time since she had returned from the hospital in mid-January. It took both of us to help her walk the short distance from the back door to the waiting car. She was bundled up—our temperatures stayed in the thirties in the day, and the snow cover persisted.
   At the doctor's office building, we turned down an offer of a wheelchair so we could give Mom some exercise. With Ginny coaching verbally, we coaxed Mom through the hallway, up the elevator, and across the hall into the doctor's office. Occasionally Mom let her feet go limp, so Ginny and I each held her up from opposite sides, our hands under her arms. "Walk, Rhoda," Ginny said. Mom smiled and told Ginny, "I am," but her legs remained limp. "No, you're not, Rhoda," Ginny said. "You've got to walk; come on, Rhoda." Eventually Mom began to move her feet, and

Ginny and I loosened our grip but remained ready to catch her as she tried to walk under her own power.

Mom weighed in at 86.2 pounds, up from eighty-five a month ago and from eighty-one at her low point. Of course we had to have four hands holding her on the scale, so we may have added a pound or so to the weight, but it was still a good sign. When Dr. Kay examined her, the redness in her eyes was gone for the first time in several days. It probably had resulted from a cold, which, miraculously, she seems to have shaken, weakened immune system and all. Dr. Kay marveled that she is doing as well as she is. She can't count back from one hundred as she did in October (I tried counting with her before the doctor arrived, and the best I could get was a smile and "You're right," as I counted back from one hundred).

When we walked into the house upon our return from the doctor's appointment, a package awaited us. It was a beautiful outfit for Mom from Millie and Mel. It was very nice of them, and Mom enjoyed the outfit and the thought that they sent it.

Saturday, March 31
Betty said to us, "You should take Rhoda out for a car ride more often. She seems so much better than she has been in two weeks, and it seems that this is all since you and Ginny took her to the doctor's." I suspected that the cold she had been fighting for two weeks had sapped her strength a bit. Also, Nicole told me this morning that the swelling in the feet seemed to be reduced significantly, so the support stockings may be working. I'll await confirmation from one of the regular caregivers because they are more familiar with Mom's condition and have monitored her feet more closely and frequently than I.

Desiree came for the late-night shift and told us that she had been fired by Med Link for working for us independently while she was an employee of theirs and, at times, being assigned here by them. She is vulnerable for a $2,500 fine in addition. She said she tried to explain that we were ready to drop Med Link entirely because our insurance was running out, and that we only continued hiring her through Med Link on Saturday nights because she,

Desiree, had urged us to. Otherwise, they would be getting no business from us.

Perhaps I am biased because Desiree is so good to Mom and the children, and her flexibility has been so valuable for us, but it sounds like she may have a boss who wants to use her as an example to others. I realize that a policy is a policy, and that Desiree violated it, but there are extenuating circumstances: when we offered Desiree several nights of work a week, we were under the impression that Mom would only be with us a few weeks, and we wanted the caregivers we knew were good with Mom for what we thought were her final days, weeks at the most.

I'm putting my advocate's hat back on and preparing a strong letter to Med Link. I will let them know that some of the people they have sent us have been incompetent, and that some of the people they had sent us were coming for an all-night shift right after completing a ten-hour shift elsewhere, and they were understandably exhausted. I'm hopeful of reversing the decision with Desiree, but she said she couldn't work for them anyway. She said she is going to enroll full time in college next semester to become a doctor and will have a difficult schedule. This may preclude working for any agency, although she could probably land a job with one of the other agencies because they are so short on personnel, and she is good.

Happily, Mom continued on an even keel. She slept ten to twelve hours a night, was alert during the day with an occasional nap, still used our names regularly, even if interchangeably, and was lots of fun to converse with at the dinner table or as she sat on the couch during the day. Clearly, she feels part of a family, as do the caregivers. We have adapted to her, and she to us, in the same way that we all adapt to each other and to our children as they advance through different stages of life. We react differently according to each other's needs and wants at a particular stage in life, but the love, the joy of being together, the humor, and the caring are no different—just the behaviors of how these are acted out.

Gary called to say that he is planning to come next Saturday and Sunday, and he asked if we are still going to be away celebrating Passover with Sue's family. I told him that we will be leaving next Saturday morning, assuming Mom's still holding her own, and returning on Monday night. He asked, "Is there anything I can do to help out while I am there at your house?" I told him, "I will leave the files out; it would be helpful if you could go through them. There are still unopened envelopes from Tower Administration, Medicare, etc. I've just been too busy to even see what bills should be paid, although I don't think I have missed anything major. There is probably about an hour's worth of opening, sorting, and reading." Gary indicated that he will be here for most of Saturday and until around four o'clock on Sunday. We agreed to talk Sunday morning, and he will call me any time if there is a problem or if he or any of the caregivers has a question.

Laurie reminisces about her mother-in-law:
The quality I admired most in her was that she was always choosing to put others first.

Raina reminisces about her grandmother:
Knowing Grandma from the time I was really young and then when she was living with us and had Alzheimer's, the quality I admired the most in her was that she never had a bad word to say about anyone.

Simone, the Incompetent Caregiver

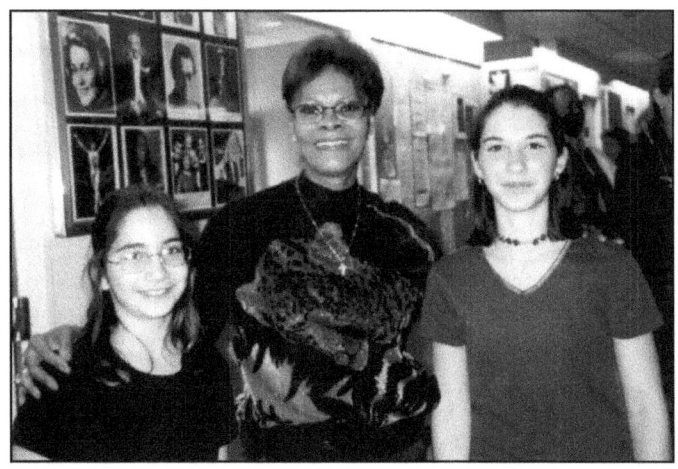

Singer Dionne Warwick with Raina
(left) and Marli, March 17, 2001

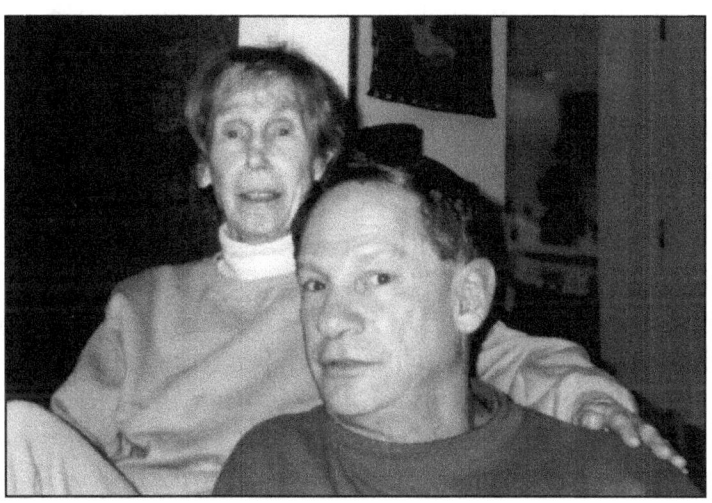

Mom and son Don near the end

Chapter 16

A Thief in Our Midst

Monday, April 2

I know it will sound crazy to be upbeat and simultaneously report a marked deterioration in her physical condition, but Mom is still such a pleasure to be with; none of what's happening is unexpected and, in fact, is slower in coming than we expected, so there's nothing for us to complain about. At Ginny's suggestion, we took the wheelchair out of hiding and made it available to all caregivers. The stress on Mom of lifting her up and down and encouraging her to walk was diminishing the value of any exercise she might have been receiving. Mom experienced back pain last night, and the caregiver administered a pain-killer—the first time in about a month.

Mom speaks more softly, tires more easily, and slides down the couch a little when she sits there, but she continues to enjoy company and talks frequently. She'll say "Don" or sometimes call me Raina or Marli, but she will ask something when she spots me at a distance and wants my attention. For instance, today I walked into the kitchen and waved from one end of the room to the family room, where she was seated. She looked up, smiled, and waved back. Then she signaled me to come over to her, which I did, and she began whispering questions.

This afternoon, Ginny called me upstairs to show me a little blood in the nose. She called the doctor, who suggested a cotton swab and some other things. Mom looked frail but so trusting and so comfortable. Also this afternoon, Ginny noticed a skin irritation on her back; she called hospice for advice on creams to use.

"How are you doing, Mom?" I asked while Ginny was on the phone.

"Fine," she said, giving no indication of whether she really understood the question. Yet, so typically, she has an affirmative response for any question put to her.

"I'm going to miss you." I said.

She got serious and responded, "I know."

"Gary will be here this weekend, and he will be with you while we take a brief trip. Can you hold out until Gary gets here?"

"Oh, sure," she said, and offered a faint smile.

I left the house long enough to drive into the village and deliver a seven-page letter to Med Link, describing our concerns with their service and strongly suggesting that I will publicly announce our discontent with them if they follow through with firing Desiree and fining her. In the letter I went into detail explaining that Desiree is one of the few competent caregivers they have sent, that we only continued using Med Link, to some degree, because of Desiree, and that our use of her privately was not in place of going through Med Link, but was because insurance coverage was about to run out. Med Link charges twice what we have to pay when we solicit caregivers privately, yet insurance won't cover us unless we go through a state-certified agency, and we often get better results when we don't go through an agency.

Wednesday, April 4

At six thirty this morning, I was downstairs at the computer, where time flies by when I am focused on my work. Mom often doesn't stir before ten or eleven, but occasionally she's up much earlier. I went upstairs at nine thirty, and I saw Ginny lifting Mom, who was in a prone position, up in bed to a sitting position and then moving her to the wheelchair. This was the first time I realized how much more help Mom needs now than even two weeks ago. Half an hour later, I once again reappeared from my cellar office; Mom was at the breakfast table. She looked up and said, "Hi, Don, how are you?"

"I'm fine, Mom, how are you?"

"Good," she answered.

"Are you taking proper care of Ginny, keeping her out of trouble?" I asked.

"Sure!"

I received a nice e-mail from Fred, once again expressing his admiration for what we are doing for Mom, and then he shared: "Things are hopping here. I can't believe how such a small commitment, like deciding to run for public office, can turn into such a big undertaking. I suspect I must have been of the same mentality that I was when I ran for student council. I can say that it is very interesting and challenges you to learn a lot in a short period of time. A city is an incredible complexity of law, politics, economics, psychology, ecology, and many other frameworks. Some I am familiar with, and others I have to learn. I knew and still know precious little about zoning and planning in a city, which turn out to be crucial, for example."

Thursday, April 5

As I entered the house from teaching my course at the university, Mom and Ginny were sitting on the couch. I saw Ginny raise her leg while Mom watched. "We're doing exercises," Ginny explained. "Only Mom's not joining me."

Ginny raised her leg again, and I raised mine. "Come on, Mom, exercise," I said.

Mom grinned a broad, happy grin, looked at me with amusement, but didn't move a muscle as Ginny and I continued to raise and lower our legs alternately.

Then Ginny lifted an arm and asked Mom to join in. Once again, Mom looked at Ginny, said "Sure," laughed, and did nothing. Finally, Ginny lifted Mom's arms for her. Mom smiled and, after much prodding, began to participate.

Nancy came by for her weekly visit. Everything is okay, except Mom's feet are swelling again. I noticed that Mom was still in the wheelchair, and I realized that she spends most of her time in that chair now when she is awake. But she's adjusted nicely.

I went out for a while, and when I returned, I found Betty and Mom at the dinner table. Mom was eating, feeding herself.

Friday, April 6

Mom got up around eleven thirty. She was cheerful as ever at the breakfast table. She ate well. Ginny kidded with her, and the two were laughing, as usual. By two thirty, Mom was napping again. We fear that she may be coming down with a cold. Gary arrives tomorrow. Flowers arrived from the Fitzgeralds, and they are gorgeous. Mom kept looking at them and smiling. "Mom," I said, "aren't they beautiful? Look at the tulips and that gorgeous lily."

"It's beautiful," Mom responded.

Gary e-mailed: "You all have done more for Mom than anyone could have asked, so it is important that Susan and the kids can be with their cousins and sibs. If I can help that process in a very small way, it is the least I can do. I had hoped to be able to stay until Monday but have to be back to testify before the General Assembly. There are to be huge budget cuts in North Carolina this year, and we will have to fight for every penny."

I responded that we were all set for him, and whatever time he can spend will be helpful. I pointed out that we have competent caregivers who will be here all the time, so he needn't stay any longer than he can afford.

"The guest room is all set for you if you want to stay at the house. I will leave the box of files on the bed in the guest room. I'll leave the checkbook to Mom's account out in case there are any bills to be paid; I think I'm on top of the few that come here. Most are being directed to you."

Diane e-mailed to say that my uncle Sam, her dad, will be having Passover at her house. She added: "We just read your e-mail. We will keep you all in our prayers. Wish we could do more to help. Let me know if there is anything we can do."

Saturday, April 13

I received a letter from Mr. O'Bryan at Med Link, apologizing profusely for their errors, assuring me that he has shared my letter with all the people at Med Link, and that there will be improvements. While he did not agree to rehire Desiree, he assured me that he would not seek to collect the $2,500 fine that was part of the penalty for working for us and Med Link at the same time. Since Desiree says she doesn't want to work for Med Link anymore, the dropping of the fine is the major thing we could have gotten out of this mess. His closing paragraph was indicative of the positive tone of his entire letter, which I appreciated:

"On a personal note, my grandmother spent three years living with my family, suffering from Alzheimer's when I was in high school. It's not the same as your situation, but I do understand the stress that is put on a family under those circumstances. Regardless of the problems we have discussed, I hope that Med Link has in some way been able to help your family. My best wishes to you. Sincerely,

Matthew O'Bryan"

Desiree wasn't available for her usual all-night Saturday shift; however, Betty arrived at five this morning and is prepared to stay twenty-six hours until seven o'clock tomorrow morning. This wouldn't have been possible a few months ago because it would have been too demanding for any caregiver. But now that Mom sleeps through, the overnight caregivers get a good night's sleep in the bed alongside of her.

Mom continued to be as alert as ever. When at the table, she'd look up at the slightest sound of someone walking behind her or of a door opening or closing. She complained of pain in her head tonight, and Sue asked if I thought we should give Mom the morphine. We agreed to wait ten minutes and see if it recurred. It didn't, and Mom seemed fine.

Sunday, April 14

At seven this morning, Nicole wasn't here on time. Betty offered to remain an extra two hours, which was twenty-eight hours in all for her. When Nicole finally arrived, she claimed that she had been in Syracuse with her daughter, and that she had called her agency to let them know that she would be late. The agency representative told us that they never received her call. Fortunately, Sundays and Wednesdays are the only times we now use an agency.

Monday, April 16

The week was happily uneventful. Mom slept from eleven to fourteen hours a night but was alert when awake; she seemed to understand some questions, and as always, she enjoyed everyone's company. She continued to feed herself, often needing coaxing or modeling.

Ginny took Mom outside to enjoy the sunshine for the first time since the trip to the doctor a couple of weeks ago. Raina found an unused five-foot plank of wood to use as a ramp, and Ginny rolled Mom's wheelchair onto our large deck off the kitchen. She seemed to really enjoy the sunshine. Just in case the beauty of the environment wasn't enough to occupy Mom, Raina and Ginny provided entertainment by having a catch until the ball rolled onto the pool cover.

Mom is now in the wheelchair all the time, except when a caregiver lifts her out of the chair and onto the couch for extended periods. All of our caregivers are strong, able to lift Mom by themselves, as they often have to do. Our four primary caregivers are all outstanding, and they have created their own telephone tree for times when they need to trade hours and cover for each other so they don't have to bother us. Previously, they would let us know if one of them needed to miss a scheduled time, and then we would try to provide coverage. Now it's so much easier because they find their own replacements when necessary.

Wednesday, April 18

Helen Lobell called to ask about Mom. She reminded me that she is two months older than Mom, and they have known each other since they were fifteen. She spoke of some of their times together and of the irony that she, Helen, is so much in control of her faculties yet at the same age as Mom. Rae Horowitz also called. She had just gotten out of the hospital, where she was treated for congestive heart failure. We put the phone to Mom's ear as Rae spoke to her.

Friday, April 20
    Shirley's Journal:
        Rhoda fed herself almost all of her meal. Outside at 2 pm, back in at 3:15. Rhoda enjoyed the sun and the wheelchair rides and watching Sue put the summer things out by the pool. Down at 3:30 pm.

Saturday, April 21

At times, Mom seems so fragile and exhausted that I don't expect her to be around by the end of the week. She has to be lifted out of bed each morning and after each nap, and she has to be lifted into bed at night. When she's not in bed, she is in the wheelchair or on the couch in the family room, and when she is in the wheelchair, she's usually at the kitchen table. She still likes to read from the headlines on a magazine or newspaper article, often aloud. Or she will read, aloud, "Rosa Parks," from the large poster board dangling from the bottom of the kitchen counter, a project Raina did this year for her fifth grade class. The last few days, we've been able to get her outside on the back deck as the weather has recently averaged above fifty degrees (above seventy today).

Today Raina took many pictures of Mom, bundled up in a winter coat with a Russian Cossack-type hat. At one point, as I worked in a garden about fifty yards away, I heard Raina saying, "Grandma, look at the camera; stop looking at your son." I turned to see Raina focusing the camera on Mom, but Mom was looking way off to the side where I was weeding. I got up from the ground and walked behind Raina and said, "Smile, Mom, for the picture." Mom looked right at me and the camera and started smiling, weakly. "Mom, you can do better than that," I said. Where's that famous smile you always told me was so important?" As I laughed, Mom opened her mouth into a weak, but friendly grin, and Raina snapped the picture.

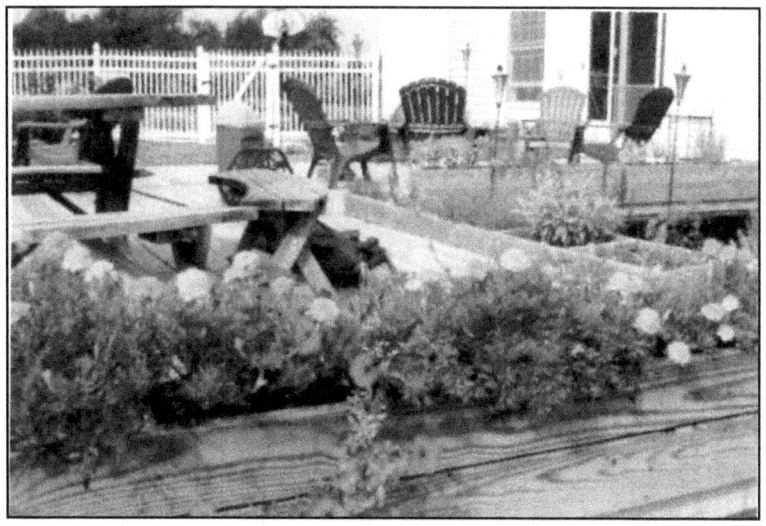

The deck outside the back kitchen door to the house was where Mom could see Don garden and the children play at a time she could no longer walk.

Today was a good day. Mom was alert as she sat outside for a while. When she was on the sofa in the family room, she often watched tapes with the caregiver, and sometimes Raina joined them. They've seen *Gypsy* a few times and *Fiddler* this past week. Marli, Sue, or I often stopped by to watch briefly with them or just to talk with Mom. Her voice is even softer now than it has been, but she still spoke audibly. She seemed to understand simple questions and responded. But it's hard to tell what she really understood or whether we asked the question more than once if we didn't get the anticipated answer the first time, which cued her that we were seeking a different response.

"Are you hungry, Rhoda?" the caregiver asked. Mom smiled and nodded.

Was she hungry, or was the question asked in a way that encouraged an affirmative response? We rarely ask a question that can't be responded to with a yes or no. Mom always seems to respond with yes, no, sure, or okay. But often her responses do seem to fit the situation.

"Ouch," I said as I got my hand too close to the stove. "What's the matter?" Mom asked, looking up. "I burned my hand," I said. "That's too bad," Mom replied, again with the appropriate words.

Mom continues to feed herself, although she often has to be reminded that there is food on her spoon or fork. She sits for a while, just holding her utensil as any or all of us mimic the routine of bringing the utensil to our mouths, or we actually eat, hoping that she will do the same.

No matter how much she deteriorates physically, two things remain constant: first, her obvious enjoyment in dialoguing with us and knowing that we are with her and that she is part of the family meals and the family goings-on; and second, her relative freedom from any pain or discomfort. She has a purple bruise mark on her forehead. We suspect that one of the agency caregivers may have dropped her or, more likely, bumped her head as they were lifting her or maneuvering her in the bathroom. The regular caregivers are very quick to let us know of any problems Mom has, and they don't fear being blamed. In fact, they will report in their journals any time Mom falls while they are on duty. Other caregivers often try to hide it if Mom has fallen during their shift. No one told us of this bruise until Ginny noticed a purple blotch on Mom's forehead. Fortunately, it doesn't seem to bother Mom and isn't getting any worse.

Each day is just so delightful when it is blessed with one of Mom's smiles—and the smiles are always easy to bring forth. What more can we ask?

Sunday, April 22

Yesterday was Gail's fiftieth birthday, and she e-mailed: "Thanks for my birthday greetings! I was lucky enough to have my birthday on a weekend, so we had a lovely time! Had a leisurely day, with a family-made lunch and a PINK birthday cake with only five candles! And John got me a really nice watch, which was a super surprise. In the evening we went en famille to see *Midsummer Night's Dream* with one of our best women comediennes playing Bottom, and we loved it. I am so sorry to hear about Aunt Rhoda getting weaker and weaker, but it is so good that she isn't in pain and is able to enjoy being with you all. Much love to all of you, and please give your mom a big hug and big hello to all of you from all of us!"

Wednesday, April 25

Susan is our big news tonight. She tried to go from the first step on the deck to the third step without using the second step. After a late-night visit to the emergency room, she now has her crutches, instructions to keep the foot elevated, and frustration that some of her activities have been limited. She has a bad sprain. I suggested that if she gets up early each morning, she could use Mom's wheelchair because Mom consistently sleeps until ten or eleven. I asked Betty if she could handle two patients for the price of one. She's still laughing, although she hasn't agreed.

Thursday, April 26

Nancy visited and observed, "I've never seen an Alzheimer's patient like your mother; she is so expressive, responds to every comment and every person." Mom spoke in a whisper, but continued to communicate.

Friday, April 27

Mom was as alert as ever. If one of us entered the house, Mom's attention wandered toward the person entering, and she kept looking until you joined her at the table or sofa—wherever she was at the time. Then she gave that big smile of greeting.

Raina has become quite proficient at crocheting, thanks to Betty's tutelage. Raina, Mom, and the caregiver will often sit on the sofa, watching a tape of *Gypsy*, or *Gigi*, or one of Raina's other favorites while Raina crochets. This afternoon, Marli left for Albany to spend the weekend participating in the state championships for speech and debate. "It's hard to believe, Mom, isn't it, that shy Marli could argue a point with anyone?" I asked. Mom offered that knowing smile and her usual shrug of the shoulders, which she characteristically gives when you suggest something ridiculous. She may not be able to process the meaning of most comments, but she does, clearly, understand what type of response is appropriate.

Saturday, April 28

Sue followed the doctor's advice and sat on the back deck all day, foot in the air, phone in her ear. She was feeling much better, although she still had some discomfort, but she hasn't needed the pain-killer since Thursday, and she is hoping to begin using an air cast soon.

Thursday, May 3

Ginny's Journal:

Rhoda sleeping when I arrived, 8 am. Waking at very short intervals, up at 10:45 am, bed bath, applied shield skin to sores on left knee area and right elbow. Rhoda had a very large red spot, left hip area. Applied A+D. Rhoda was very soaked this am so that is probably how the red spot started. I applied Gold Bond powder. We went outside, and I pushed her wheelchair around the property so she could enjoy the flowers. Daffodils, tulips, and hyacinths, in abundance, are in full bloom.

Sunday, May 6

Mom kept leaning forward and trying to get out of the wheelchair today. We think this is because of sore areas where she sits, despite an array of ointments and the frequent turning done to Mom by the caregivers.

We think we've figured out why Mom awakens each morning calling everyone Raina. There is a picture by her bed that Raina drew and signed for Mom. Ginny pointed out that when she turns Mom to the left in the morning, Mom is facing the picture, which is signed, "I love you, Raina."

As I reflect back to last October when Mom came to live with us, the deterioration, physically, has been continual. It is more like she is going slowly and quietly but remaining the essence of herself to the end. Jennifer came by from hospice and observed, "I'll bet she was a very social person, always striking up conversations with whoever was around."

How long can she hang in there? Each week, I wonder if she can go another. But the personality is there, even if the physical abilities continue to decline.

Monday, May 7
Betty is the caregiver whose shift ends at eight in the morning, and she told me half an hour before she left that last night Mom needed a small dose of pain medication. Betty said, "She kept whispering, 'Help me,' and seemed to be in discomfort, having difficulty sleeping." According to Betty, once given the morphine, Mom went right to sleep and was still sleeping then at 7:45 a.m.

Ginny took over, and after Mom was awake and in the family room, Ginny asked, "Rhoda, how many banana slices are in your bowl?" Mom smiled and nodded. Three times Ginny repeated the question. Finally Mom whispered, "Four." She was right.

While barely speaking even in a whisper, Mom continued to be alert. She motioned me to come near her. I walked across the family room, knelt beside her, put my hand on hers, and said, "How are you doing?"

She shrugged and spoke inaudibly.

"I wish I could understand what you are saying," I responded, more candidly than usual.

Mom gave a faint smile and shrugged again.

There are other signs of deterioration: longer sleeping, more times when she is agitated—possibly due to sores on the rear—probably a little weight loss, a total inability to lift herself up or walk, even with help, and an inability to move from whatever spot she is placed in. But she keeps smiling and reacting.

Saturday, May 12

We have what may be a disturbing development that has nothing to do with Mom. I think someone may be taking money from the envelope in my dresser where I keep the cash to pay the caregivers. I keep careful records of how much money we are paying each caregiver, but I have not kept an accurate accounting of how much money I put in the envelope every few weeks. None of the caregivers has cause to be in our bedroom, and the only other person who is ever there is a woman who has been cleaning our house every two weeks for a few years. She lives down the road, and we are sure she wouldn't take money from us.

This morning I opened the drawer of my bedroom dresser to get the cash to pay Ginny, and it appeared to me that there might be less money in the envelope than there should be. But I am not sure. We have so many caregivers—some putting in a full week of work, and others coming for just a day or an evening each week—that it's possible the money is being drained more quickly than I think. If someone is taking money from the drawer, they are being careful not to take too much at a time because there always seems to be a reasonable amount of money there, unless it has been a while since my last trip to the bank, in which case I don't expect to have much cash in the envelope.

Today, for the first time, I counted the amount of money in the drawer, recorded it, and put the paper in a file in a cabinet in my basement office. I am hoping there will be nothing missing as I begin to keep track. All of the caregivers we have had recently appear to be trustworthy.

Sunday, May 13

Diane e-mailed: "This must be a bittersweet Mother's Day for you and Gary. I am glad Rhoda is still giving you joy. Spent last week with Dad; he is amazing, somewhat repetitive, but still very active. We are lucky to still have him. Thinking of all of you, Diane."

Mother's Day is nice. Sue, Marli, Raina, and I traveled forty-five minutes into Canada to have an early brunch buffet at one of our favorite restaurants. Long-stemmed red roses were a gift to all the mothers. We returned home around two o'clock and walked in the door to the family room shortly after Mom had awakened. She was sitting on the couch, ready to greet us, having heard the car coming up the driveway, and probably also getting a clue from Frisky's barking. Sue handed Mom her rose and said, "Happy Mother's Day, Mom!" Mom's face brightened with a broad smile that demonstrated her appreciation and, possibly, her understanding.

After a few hours of family gardening, we brought in Italian food for Raina and Indian for Marli, Sue, and me. Joann, from the agency, sat with Mom on the couch while we ate a few yards away in the kitchen. It was only Joann's second time here. She seemed nice, but she was awfully quiet. Marli said, "Joann, I think Grandma wants you to talk to her; she's talking to you."

"I am," said Joann, "very quietly." Well, it's doubtful that Joann had said anything for the past hour, so Marli silently mouthed a comment about Joann to the rest of us, which wasn't intended to compliment Joann on her smarts. Joann did lighten our day after dinner. She told us that when we put the Italian and Indian food on the table, Mom turned to her and commented: "Something smells. In fact, it stinks!" Before I left the kitchen to go downstairs to check my e-mail, I went over to Mom and said: "You've had a good day, Mom. While I'm sorry you didn't like the aroma of our dinner, we did enjoy it." Mom smiled and lifted both hands, palms up, with the shrug that is so typical of her. Does this mean she understood the gist of what I had just said? Why else would she raise her palms upward in a shrug?

At seven fifty, Shirley arrived and probably said more to Mom during a three-minute greeting than Joann had spoken the previous five hours. Mom was still enjoying Shirley's company as I prepared to turn in.

Thursday, May 17

Twice in the past ten days, Mom has slept from ten at night until four or five the next afternoon. She still speaks barely loud enough to be heard and rarely coherently for more than a sentence. But she remains keenly aware of who is around her and what is happening. Again, she was able to identify the number of objects Ginny was pointing to.

Twice in the past four days, Mom went more than twenty-four hours without urinating. Nancy came late this afternoon, prepared to insert a catheter. Sue was in the kitchen when Nancy and Ginny went into Mom's room, catheter in hand. A moment later, Nancy emerged and said to Sue, "She's gone." Sue turned pale, assuming the worst. "No," said Nancy, "I didn't mean that. I meant she's gone to the bathroom." We all got a good laugh at that later on, when Mom was clearly in good spirits and doing well. Mom was able to go just in time so that the catheter was averted. However, Nancy did say that the lengthy sleeps, the infrequency of urination, and a few other signs could indicate that the end is a matter of days. She hastened to add that, as when they gave us a maximum of four weeks in January, there are times when someone lives for much longer.

We've come a long way as a family since October, and the routine for all of us has been changed drastically; it has taken some major adjustments. Now we've made the adjustments. Another round of changes in our routines when, inevitably, we lose Mom, will be even more difficult than the ones we have made since last October.

Mom continued to be alert when she was awake or at the dinner table with us. She is so thin that she once actually slid out of the wheelchair. The caregivers have had to adapt too; Betty made a belt/bib, which holds Mom in the chair.

Mom feeds herself with prodding from Raina and Sue most of the time and occasionally from Marli or me. Initially Mom will hold her spoon in her hand, with food on it, or look at one of us, enjoying the camaraderie. "Eat, Mom," someone will say. Mom will smile, look at the person talking, but do nothing to lift the utensil toward her mouth. Then the coaxing, cajoling, and strategizing will begin.

Kim, a caregiver from the agency, did a decent job, but not of the caliber of the private caregivers. Sue asked her nicely, "Please encourage Mom to feed herself. She can do it. Can't you, Mom?" Kim put the fork in Mom's hand as Sue coached. "Mom, show Kim you can feed yourself," Sue pleaded. Mom smiled and looked at Sue.

"Come on, Mom," Sue continued, as we all began to mimic taking the fork and putting food in our mouths. After smiling and staring at us for a few minutes, Mom finally lifted the food to her mouth and ate as Kim watched with amazement. "I guess she can do it," Kim said, and then she began coaxing Mom as she saw Sue do. We may have only a few days left. But then again, that's what we thought last January.

Gary and I talked, and he told me that he hopes the prediction that Mom may have only a few days is as accurate as the one in January.

Saturday, May 19

Each day, I count the money I put in the envelope in our bedroom drawer, and I record any amount I take from the envelope to pay caregivers. Four hundred dollars disappeared from the envelope between eight this morning and three this afternoon. Only Betty and Desiree and the lady who cleans have been in the house. I am certain that Betty could not possibly have taken the money, and I doubt very much it is Desiree, but I really don't believe the woman who cleaned for us could be guilty of this either. Yet I was so sure it was neither Betty nor Desiree that I was tempted to suspect the woman who cleans, just by process of elimination. But Susan was just as sure that it couldn't be her.

Sue and I went to a police officer who is also a friend and the parent of one of Raina's classmates. He referred us to a private investigator, who set up a surveillance camera disguised as a smoke detector in a part of the ceiling where a detector could have been.

We plan to drive Marli to Norwood Tuesday night—half an hour from our home—where she is to play her cello with the school's orchestra in a musical production. Norwood-Norfolk is a small school district and apparently needs a cello player for its annual show. Desiree will be on duty Tuesday night, and I am sure she isn't the thief, but just in case, I am going to set a trap.

Monday, May 21

I was planting lavender petunias, orange celosia, and yellow marigolds in a garden in the pool area when I heard Ginny knock on the window and point me out to Mom, who was seated at the kitchen table. Mom looked out the picture window at me, and when I waved to her, she lifted her arm and waved back. This may not sound like much, but these days, any movement for Mom is an effort.

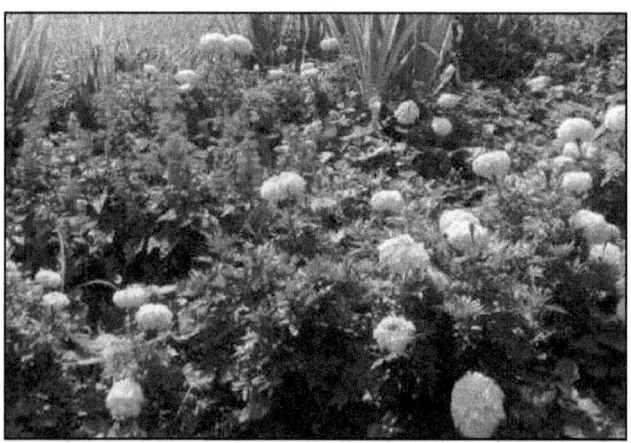

Yellow marigolds and red salvia dominate one of the many gardens. Mom loved color.

These last few days have seen improvement. Mom is more alert. She waves when one of us waves to her. She speaks less frequently, and when she does, it is not loud enough to be heard by an ear more than a few inches from her mouth. Yet she still has responded coherently to each of us several times in the past two days.

Gary called and asked if we thought we would be able to attend Todd's wedding to Katie over Memorial Day weekend in Minneapolis. I told him that we really hadn't thought about not attending since the doctor's prognosis in January made it seem definite that Mom wouldn't be with us anywhere near Memorial Day. Sue and I will discuss it tonight, and we'll also see how Mom is as the week progresses. Right now she seems good for at least a week, but any day something is possible.

After lunch Ginny and Mom watched a video with Raina and me in it; also they watched a little of the *Fantasia* video and looked through picture albums. Mom was alert and more talkative today than she has been recently, although still difficult to hear.

Tuesday, May 22

We had an early dinner, and as we prepared to leave for the show in Norwood, I told Desiree that we would call when it was over to see how Mom is doing. I wanted her to be confident that we wouldn't walk in on her until at least half an hour after she had received a call from us.

I counted the money in the dresser drawer carefully before we left, and I made sure there were several thousand dollars so that Desiree—if she is the thief—will think that she can take a few hundred dollars without it being noticed. When we came back from the concert, another four hundred dollars was missing. It was Desiree. The P.I. will probably not be able to come for the tape and show it to us until late tomorrow afternoon. We will report her to the police as soon as we have the tape and incontrovertible evidence it is her.

We are hoping to have everything involving the theft worked out by tomorrow, and if Mom is okay this week, we'll all be attending the wedding on Saturday. We are packing and getting ready to go.

Wednesday, May 23

The video of Desiree taking the money did not come out. Either I hadn't heard correctly or the P.I. forgot to mention that I needed to leave a light on somewhere in or near the room for the video to work. The P.I. showed us how to view the video so we won't have to go to him in the future if we have another opportunity to capture the theft on camera. Desiree is scheduled to work this weekend. We're still hoping that we might be able to travel to Minnesota for the wedding. If we are, I will set the camera up with a nearby light on this time.

Mom hasn't gotten out of bed today; she has awakened only briefly for a few minutes, a few times. Betty took over for Ginny at four o'clock, and at six she asked me if Ginny had called hospice. Betty said she thinks that some of the signs might be here that we are near the end. I said, "Mom was really alert yesterday," but Betty said, "That's one of the signs." Betty called hospice, and Nancy said she'd send Barbara over if we wanted. I indicated that she should come. Our plane was scheduled to leave Friday evening for Minnesota and Todd and Katie's wedding. If necessary, I will stay back and encourage Susan, Marli, and Raina to go. Darren is scheduled to meet us Saturday in Minnesota, flying in from Flagstaff.

Barbara arrived and went directly upstairs to check on Mom. Barbara had been here for an hour and was still examining her. Mom's arm was too thin for Barbara to take her blood pressure. She has been unable to take fluids since yesterday. Betty kept giving her the special liquid lollipop for some fluid. Barbara said that if Mom can't take fluids, she wouldn't have more than a few days. I know Ginny will do everything possible tomorrow to get Mom to sit up and take fluids, so we'll find out then.

Barbara told me—after completing a thorough examination—that Mom's passing isn't imminent, but if she were me she wouldn't go away for more than three days. "We will be able to tell a lot more in the morning," she said. She also said that she will send over a hospital bed so Mom wouldn't have to be lifted as often.

While Mom was awake in bed, I held her hand and looked in her eyes. She managed a smile, tried whispering something to me a few times, and we continued to hold hands. She seemed pain free and oh so peaceful. Betty relies on gestures from Mom for communication, and she told me Mom felt warm—but was cold.

"How do you know?" I asked. "Because she keeps pulling up her blanket. When she moves her arms from side to side, she wants to be turned. When she raises her hand to her mouth, she wants a drink."

Thursday, May 24

Mom was a little better this morning. With the help of the hospital bed rolling her up to a near sitting position, Ginny was able to get her to sit up long enough to eat some yogurt and drink some water. We'll see how she is later today. We may ask the nurse from hospice to return. We can leave as late as four o'clock tomorrow afternoon and still make the plane with ease. It's eleven thirty now, and Mom is looking as she did earlier in the week. Susan and I are on our way to see the sheriff to brief him on our suspicions and our plans to try the camera again; also we have asked Nancy to come over and look at Mom. We will make a decision on travel soon.

I called Gary and brought him up-to-date. He said, "Obviously we would love to see all of you but will understand whatever you decide to do."

Friday, May 25

By noon Mom was much improved, so we prepared to leave, hoping we can still attend the wedding. Once again I counted the money carefully, but this time I left on a small light near the fish tank at the opposite end of the room from our bed. I also left a note downstairs for all caregivers who will watch Mom in our absence, asking them to leave the small bedroom light on because it is necessary, I said, for the fish tank to function effectively. This was the best I could think of. There is also a tiny red light that is part of the camera, and I tried to camouflage it as much as possible. The camera, installed by the P.I., remains on the ceiling, disguised as a smoke detector.

We cut it close, making it to the airport in time for our flight. I actually made the decision to go to the wedding when we arrived at the Syracuse airport, and I called Ginny, and she said that Mom is doing okay.

Saturday, May 26

The wedding and all the festivities surrounding it were exciting and were expertly planned and executed by Katie and Todd. Each call home revealed that Mom was having a typical day—much sleep, but getting up to eat and drink, watch television, and leaf through whatever literature has been left on the kitchen table or in the family room.

Sunday, May 27

When we arrived home from the wedding at around eleven tonight, Raina went right into Mom's room, where Mom was lying awake. Shirley reported that when Raina entered her room, Mom just lit up when she saw her. "As each of you come into the room," Shirley said, "your mom just brightens and smiles joyfully." While Raina raced for Grandma's room, I immediately ran upstairs to grab the camera. It showed Desiree walking into our room and initially going to the far end of our bed, away from the drawer with the money; she may have been checking for a camera. Then she walked toward the dresser, opened the second drawer, and started to reach for the money. However, as she was reaching, she glanced toward the ceiling, apparently noticed the red light, closed the drawer without taking anything, and left the room.

Clearly, Desiree is the thief, but the proof is less than perfect. I decide to bluff. Desiree is scheduled to arrive for duty at six o'clock the next night.

Monday, May 28

I called Betty, who was scheduled to work until six tonight. It is Memorial Day, so Ginny has the day off, and Betty was scheduled to work in her stead. I informed Betty of Desiree's thievery because I don't want to catch her by surprise when I confront Desiree. I also called Shirley and asked if she could take Desiree's place for the 6:00 p.m. to 6:00 a.m. shift, and I asked her to arrive at 5:45 p.m. I described for her what has happened, and that I am going to confront Desiree at six and need her here to take over.

Shirley arrived on schedule and immediately went into the room where Mom was staying and closed the door so it would appear that Mom was sleeping. If Desiree asked, Sue would say that Marli or Raina was in there with Mom. Betty and Susan were in the kitchen giving a good imitation of loading or unloading the dishwasher while Raina and Marli waited upstairs in their bedrooms. Susan admitted later that she was shaking as it got close to six and she anticipated Desiree's momentary arrival.

Our plan was for Susan to tell Desiree that I was upstairs, and that I wanted to pay her for last week since we were in Minnesota at the time we would usually have paid her. If she asked why I wanted her to go upstairs, Susan was to say that I was exhausted and was going through papers and would prefer not to have to interrupt my work to go downstairs.

Desiree entered the house before six and immediately asked why there was a second car in the driveway. Susan thought quickly and explained that one of my St. Lawrence students was in the basement doing some typing for me on my computer. This would sound credible to Desiree because students have been to the house to do work for me on several occasions when she was here with Mom.

Her question answered, Desiree came up the stairs and turned left into our bedroom. Without wasting any time, I said to Desiree, "We know you've been taking money. That is not a smoke detector." I pointed toward the ceiling. "That is a camera, and we have seen you take money on several occasions, including the night of Marli's concert." Desiree immediately broke down in tears and confessed. I told her that the police would be in touch with her the next day, and I asked her to leave.

This is Desiree, the one I had saved from a $2,500 fine by sending a strong letter to her boss. This is Desiree, who had sent flowers to Marli the night of her performance in the musical revue—obviously using our money to send the flowers—and who had been doing other things to ingratiate herself to the family, such as bringing over tapes of current movies and encouraging us to keep them until we viewed them. This is Desiree, who had asked my advice about courses to take in college and to whom I had responded with half an hour of suggestions. Whether this was all an act to put herself in a position to rob us or whether she is just sick and insecure and simultaneously wanted to take the money and be liked by us is anyone's guess.

We subsequently learned that Desiree was only taking one course at the state college. The police informed us that Desiree's father is a doctor living in Phoenix, and her siblings are also successful in the field of medicine. But Desiree is apparently as far from earning a medical degree as I am, and I haven't taken a science course since I graduated from high school. Desiree's parents immediately flew from Phoenix to the North Country and sent us the $3,700 that we estimated Desiree has stolen over a period of four months. The police assured us our input will be sought before a plea bargain will be offered, but we never heard from them.

Raina took it the hardest that night after we confronted Desiree and she admitted she had stolen the money. Raina struggled to understand why. Darren wasn't caught totally off guard. He said Desiree's late-night conversations and her gifts and efforts to ingratiate herself to Darren, Marli, and Raina seemed to be too much of an effort to impress.

Approximately four years later, Sue and Raina were shopping in a nearby Walmart and were directed to a sales clerk when they asked where to find materials for a school project. The sales clerk pointed them toward the appropriate department, and as they walked away from her, Sue confirmed what Raina, who had been ten at the time of the theft, suspected—a clerk at a nearby checkout counter was Desiree.

Gary is due for a visit this Sunday. Barring the unexpected, which we are aware can happen at any time, Mom should be awake for at least part of Gary's visit and able to continue shining on all of us with the sunshine of her smile and disposition.

Tuesday, May 29

Ginny woke Mom in the morning and had her at the table, eating and drinking, when Nancy came to check her out. Mom looked and acted as she does on her better days. Nancy said that this is to be expected. Mom will have extended times of sleep, lack of drinking, and other symptoms, but will bounce back. As time goes by, there will be less bouncing back and more extended times with lack of eating and drinking.

Betty took over for Ginny late in the afternoon. Mom was eating when she arrived. She went for an indoor ride in her wheelchair, with Raina pushing. Then Raina, Betty, and Mom sat on the sofa. Mom was very tired, and Betty put her to bed at six o'clock.

I received this e-mail from Diane: "So glad that everything went well for the wedding. Sorry to learn, from Gary, about the thief! I guess you are all learning enough to write a book; in fact, Don, your 'updates' are so well written that you really should think about turning them into a book. I am sure lots of other families are now on or will face this same 'journey,' and your insights would help and reassure others. Later, when there is time, think about it."

Gary also sent an e-mail: "Thanks for the update and nice to hear Mom held her own over the weekend. Thanks also for taking the trouble to join us for the wedding. It was wonderful for us to have you all there to share our joy." He added that he would try to come to Potsdam for a quick, twenty-four-hour visit, arriving sometime on Sunday.

Susan reminisces about her mother-in-law:
I recall Mom's smile when I handed her the flower on Mother's Day, her grin when I would return from a day at school and she and Ginny would be sitting in the family room.

Diane reminisces about her aunt:
She was always sweet and joyful.

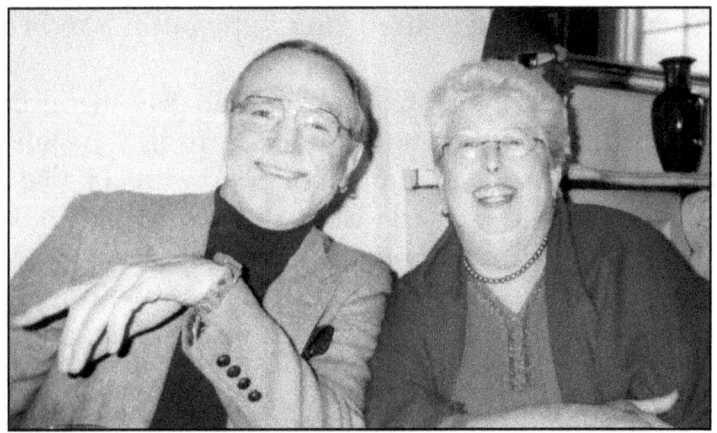

Marge and Pat Flynn: "In our faith the image comes to mind of sprinkling holy water. Now she lives in all your hearts."

Chapter 17

Grandma, These Flowers Are for You

Wednesday, May 30
Ginny's Journal:
Rhoda sleeping—waking a little at 7:15 am. Raina was off to school and telling her grandma "Bye-bye." Rhoda did a lot of reading cards and papers on the table today. Alert and talkative this afternoon. A lot of riding in the wheelchair, observing things around the house.

Sunday, June 3
Mom was resting comfortably, sitting up on the hospital bed that Barbara had sent to our home from hospice a few weeks earlier, when she began having difficulty lifting herself from a prone position.

Sue's mom, Ruth, who is eighty-one, is with us after returning to New York from her winter retirement condominium in Pompano Beach. Since the hectic pace of the past nine months had precluded us from taking our annual trip to Florida, she came to Potsdam earlier in the week for a visit. Mom experienced some discomfort in late afternoon, and Betty gave her oxygen, which provided relief.

Gary arrived this afternoon. Mom knew he was here; they had some time together before the final decline set in this evening. Betty confirmed what we were all sensing: it could be a matter of hours, maybe only minutes. Near the end, Gary and I both said, "I love you, Mom." "I love you too," she said, clearly audible.

At nine thirty tonight, Marli and Raina sneaked out of the house, flashlights in hand, and toured our gardens. They returned with a beautiful selection of flowers that they put in two vases and placed on the table near Mom's bedside. It was Marli's suggestion that they pick the flowers in order to protect Raina from seeing Grandma when she passed, but Grandma was alive when they returned, even though her eyes were about to close for the last time. As they placed the vases on the table, Raina said, "These are for you, Grandma." Grandma nodded and smiled one last somewhat-forced, but beautiful smile. Mom passed quietly at 10:19 p.m.—peacefully and with no discomfort—just twenty-five days shy of her eighty-fourth birthday.

It is fitting that Ruth was in the room at the end. The most important thing in her life had always been family, and she and my late father-in-law modeled and passed along that value to all three of their daughters. It was Susan who had pressed for years for us to build an addition to the house and to urge Mom and Ed to live with us, and then when Ed passed, to have Mom spend her remaining time with us.

Sue speculated that Mom held out until most of the family was there, and that the presence of Sue's mother, Ruth, represented someone to continue family traditions and gave Mom permission to let go. Were it not for Sue's insistence and persistence, our family would not have experienced the joy and reminders of what's important in life. That was Mom's final lesson to us all.

Monday, June 4

The funeral will be at the Levitt-Weinstein funeral home in West Palm Beach, Florida, at ten o'clock on Wednesday, which is the soonest time we can expect to have the autopsy completed and Mom's body flown to Florida. Burial is at the Eternal Light Cemetery. We are trying to arrange for a gathering place following the funeral. Our plan is to fly to Florida tomorrow morning for arrival in Ft. Lauderdale at eleven. We will meet Gary at the funeral home at one to make final arrangements and then use the afternoon to tend to details. We sent relevant information out on my group e-mail and closed with, "Our love to all of you and our thanks for all your support, communications, and understanding."

Wednesday, June 6

The funeral was a wonderful celebration of Mom's life. Gary, Laurie, Sue, Darren, Marli, Raina, Millie, Mel, Dee, Larry, and Susan's aunt Gloria were present. The rabbi conducted an informal service with some discussion. Gary and I each spoke. As if I were conducting a workshop, I asked everyone to share what they felt was Mom's most memorable characteristic. Darren said it was her positive attitude toward everything, and Marli cited her interest in others: "Grandma would always listen to me and would never say 'Now I have to go see the grown-ups.'" Raina said it was her love of colors, and Sue mentioned her interest in others as well: "She would listen over the phone with interest as Darren or Marli played the piano." Gary said he will always think of her emphasis on "the journey" and the importance of being a good sport, and I referred to Mom's focus on the importance of a smile. Mel said she always treated everyone with respect, and Millie praised her for being a caring sister. Gloria remembered how pleasant she was to everyone, and Laurie praised Mom for accepting her sons' choices of wives as her own.

Thursday, June 7

Darren left Florida for Potsdam in the Oldsmobile that had belonged to Mom and Ed since 1993, and we headed to the airport for our flights home. He asked us for a phone number for the Fitzgeralds. He wanted to break up his trip with a quick visit to see them since he has never met them but has shared in receipt of their e-mails and feels like he knows them. Through the phone conversations and exchanges of e-mails over the past eight months, the Fitzgeralds have made a strong impression on our children. Marli said to us a month ago, "We have to visit the Fitzgeralds. They sound so nice."

Friday, June 8

We arrived home from Florida, and there was an e-mail sent by Gail a few days ago: "Your mom was really special. My mom said the service was lovely, and she was so pleased that you spent time with her. It made a big difference to her, and she felt really supported by you all. Perhaps you are feeling a mixture of relief for your mom and real sadness, but you can surely feel that your mom had the kind of end that would make her feel good about her life and about those whom she had left behind. I will try phoning you over the weekend. Lots of love to all of you, Gail."

Saturday, June 9

Gary called to tell us that Darren spent the night with him and Laurie after staying with the Fitzgeralds on Thursday. He said: "It is a pleasure having Darren around, so I understand why you all enjoy it so much when he visits. Hope you all had a good trip back."

Sunday, June 10

Darren arrived in Potsdam at five. We had a pizza dinner, and then Darren announced that he found something in the car that he feels is reflective of Grandpa's personality. He produced one of Grandpa's trademark flyswatters. How fondly we recalled Grandpa's efforts to swat flies on breezy, warm summer days outdoors, as the rest of the family would sit, play by the pool, or swim.

Monday, June 11

We received an e-mail from Marge and Pat Flynn, two valued colleagues and cherished friends. Pat is my closest collaborator on workshops, on articles, and in planning and conducting the week-long summer conference of which he and I are cofounders. He and Marge and Sue and I are frequent dinner companions. He wrote: "We were saddened to learn of your mother's passing. It was our great pleasure to have known her. Her sweet, understanding nature was so obviously the wellspring of your own. Your children's closeness to her and the understanding she developed through her natural kindness is in a way one of your mother's last blessings. In my faith, the image comes to mind of a sprinkling of holy water. Now she lives in all your hearts. The older I get, the more I think of my parents, and the more I savor who they were and what they did and how they reverenced the gift of life. A mother's love makes a man. Our best to Susan, Darren, Marli, and Raina. Affectionately, Pat and Marge."

Tuesday, June 26
We received the coroner's report confirming that Mom had Alzheimer's.

Seven Years Later, an e-mail from Gary
May 24, 2008
Hi Don,

I am in Scotland today and will be working here all week and then seeing Gail and family Saturday before returning home. I keep meaning to write to you about this every time I am here but always forget. This time it is on my mind again, however, and I have a computer nearby, so here it is: I really like Scotland because it is very pretty, and the people are so friendly. Every time I am here, I think of Mom because it is the only place that rises to her level of friendliness. We used to joke about her coming out of the ladies' room with a new friend each time we stopped on a trip, and that is typical of what happens to me here. I only landed about two hours ago, and I had a long and friendly chat with the taxi driver and now with the person working at Starbucks, where I am using their wireless.

Mom would sure feel at home here, though she would probably not get very far in her sightseeing because of all of her new friends distracting her. I wonder if we had some relatives on Mom's side from Scotland?

Love, Gary

Reminiscences:
If you were able to sum up who Rhoda Mesibov (Rhoda Meister) was in one word or phrase, what would it be?

Raina:	Happy
Marli:	Gentle
Darren:	Warm
Todd:	Multifaceted
Brian:	Delightful
Gail:	Kind
Laurie:	Good sport
Gary:	Pleasant, empathetic
Susan:	Gentle
Don:	What a mother should be—unconditionally loving

Postscripts:
Susan's aunt Hazel passed away October 15, 2001, after what was described in her obituary as "too many years as an Alzheimer's patient."

Uncle Sam Alexander passed away in the home of his daughter, my cousin Diane, on February 16, 2009, a few weeks after celebrating his ninety-fifth birthday. He was officially diagnosed with age-related dementia. While some of his behaviors mimicked those of people who are officially classified as having had Alzheimer's, not all the symptoms of an Alzheimer's sufferer were present, and there was no autopsy.

Several years after Mom passed, Fred and Carole placed Aunt Mille in an assisted living home a few miles from their home in Laramie. She passed away, suffering from Alzheimer's, on March 13, 2009.

Also within a few years of Mom's passing, I had my annual physical with Dr. Kay. He told me that he would be retiring the following month because he was becoming too forgetful to continue his practice. Recently, we learned through friends that Dr. Kay is an Alzheimer's sufferer.

November 29, 2013:

Susan and I were sipping coffee and chai tea, enjoying oatmeal and a croissant at our favorite breakfast restaurant, First Crush. A gentleman—probably in his sixties or seventies—entered, accompanied by his wife, who was once a vibrant and out-going secretary at the school where Susan taught for eighteen years. He pulled the chair out for his wife, sat down next to her, smiled, and gave her an affectionate pinch on the chin. They come here often in the mornings, and the wife, as she does each time, smiled frequently but did not utter a word. She did not even nod in acknowledgement as Sue offered a warm hello.

When the server brought their pastries to the table, the husband carved hers into bite-size pieces. Susan whispered to me, "Her condition continues to deteriorate."

Is there a family as yet untouched by someone with Alzheimer's? If so, for how long?

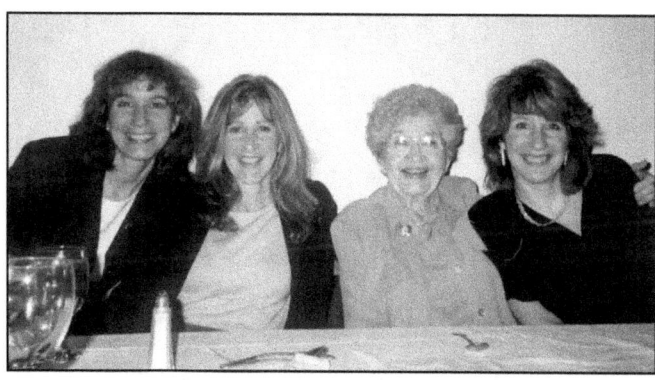

Susan's mother, Ruth, the matriarch of the family and currently ninety-four years old (2014) has always placed the importance of family above all else. Here she is shown with her three children: Cookie, Alice, and Susan.

Appreciating Mom Through the Lens of Alzheimer's

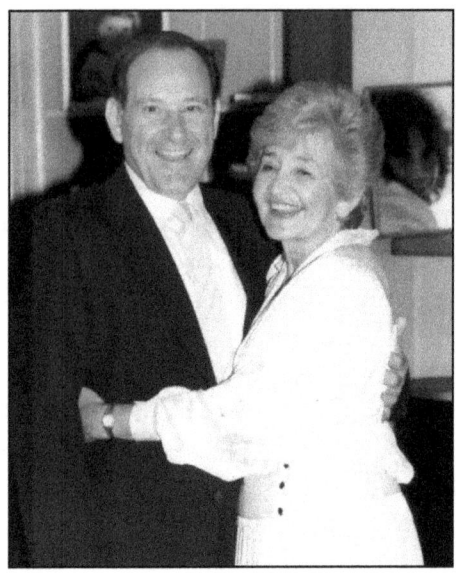

Susan's mother, Ruth, with her father, Arthur Herman, who worked for the Federal Government and served as a judge on the National Labor Relations Board. He passed away November 28, 1992.

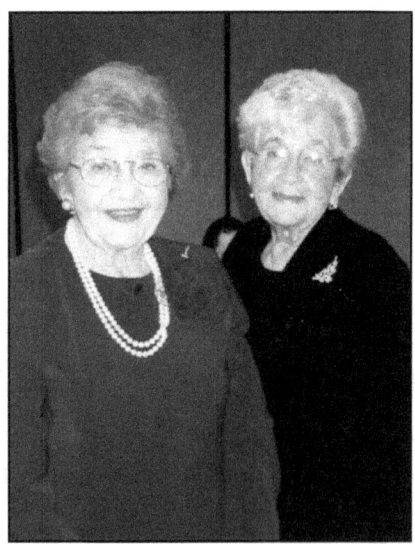

Susan's mother with her sister, Susan's Aunt Gloria.

Grandma, These Flowers Are for You

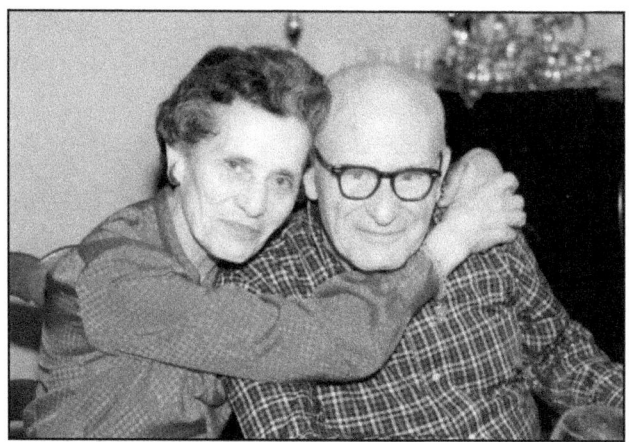

Susan's Uncle Irving, her father's brother, who also served as a judge on the National Labor Relations Board and lived until 2013, when he died at the age of ninety-nine of natural causes. Aunt Hazel died as an Alzheimer's sufferer when she was eighty-four. She spent her last years unable to communicate or to move from a prone position in her hospital bed. An excerpt from her obituary said "A generous friend to many, died October 15, 2001 after too many years as an Alzheimer's patient.

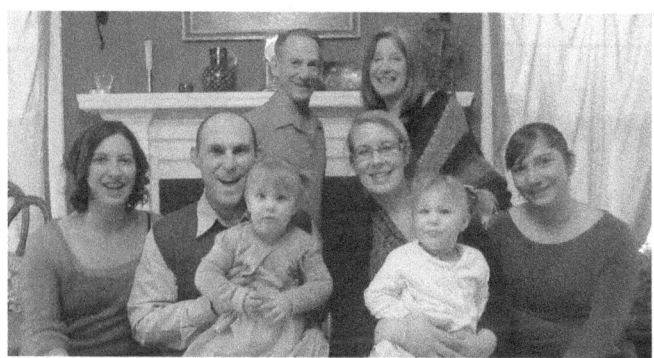

More than a decade after Mom's passing, Susan and Don, (top row); Marli (left), with Darren and Molly holding identical twin daughters; Raina (right).

Appreciating Mom Through the Lens of Alzheimer's

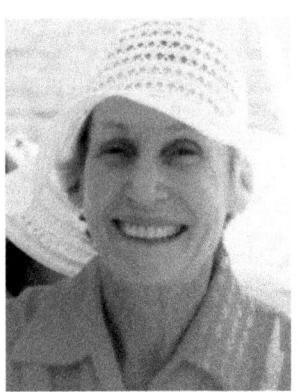

Mom, mid-1980s; long before the chilling effect of Alzheimer's began to take its toll.

www.ingramcontent.com/pod-product-compliance
Lightning Source LLC
Chambersburg PA
CBHW051636170526
45167CB00001B/211